PERINATAL MORTALITY IN NEW YORK CITY

Perinatal Mortality in New York City

RESPONSIBLE FACTORS

A STUDY OF 955 DEATHS BY
THE SUBCOMMITTEE ON NEONATAL MORTALITY,
COMMITTEE ON PUBLIC HEALTH RELATIONS,
THE NEW YORK ACADEMY OF MEDICINE,
ANALYZED AND REPORTED BY

Schuyler G. Kohl, M.S., M.D., Dr.P.H.

Published for The Commonwealth Fund
By Harvard University Press
CAMBRIDGE, MASSACHUSETTS, 1955

Published for The Commonwealth Fund
By Harvard University Press

Distributed in Great Britain
By Geoffrey Cumberlege
Oxford University Press, London

For approximately a quarter of a century THE COMMONWEALTH FUND, through its Division of Publications, sponsored, edited, produced, and distributed books and pamphlets germane to its purposes and operations as a philanthropic foundation. On July 1, 1951, the Fund entered into an arrangement by which HARVARD UNIVERSITY PRESS became the publisher of Commonwealth Fund books, assuming responsibility for their production and distribution. The Fund continues to sponsor and edit its books, and cooperates with the Press in all phases of manufacture and distribution.

MANUFACTURED IN THE UNITED STATES OF AMERICA
LIBRARY OF CONGRESS CATALOG CARD NO. 55-8999

COMMITTEE ON PUBLIC HEALTH RELATIONS

THE NEW YORK ACADEMY OF MEDICINE

1954

Harry S. Mustard, M.D., *Chairman*
Milton J. Goodfriend, M.D., *Vice Chairman*

Philip D. Allen, M.D.
J. Burns Amberson, M.D.
George E. Anderson, M.D.
Henry Aranow, Jr., M.D.
George Baehr, M.D.
Frederick R. Bailey, M.D.
Conrad Berens, M.D.
Beatrice Bishop Berle, M.D.
Carl Binger, M.D.
Linn J. Boyd, M.D.
McKeen Cattell, M.D.
C. G. deGutiérrez-Mahoney, M.D.
Haven Emerson, M.D.
José M. Ferrer, Jr., M.D.
Alfred E. Fischer, M.D.
Arthur A. Fischl, M.D.
L. Whittington Gorham, M.D.
Alan F. Guttmacher, M.D.
Hubert S. Howe, M.D.
Oswald R. Jones, M.D.
Lawrence C. Kolb, M.D.
Shepard Krech, M.D.
Asa L. Lincoln, M.D.
Harvey B. Matthews, M.D.
Fred A. Mettler, M.D.
Harry Most, M.D.
Howard A. Patterson, M.D.
Norman Plummer, M.D.
Dickinson W. Richards, M.D.
Conrad M. Riley, M.D.
Paul B. Sheldon, M.D.
Beverly C. Smith, M.D.
J. Murray Steele, M.D.
Philip M. Stimson, M.D.
Marion B. Sulzberger, M.D.
Maximin DeM. Touart, M.D.
George M. Wheatley, M.D.
I. Ogden Woodruff, M.D.
George W. Kosmak, M.D., *Emeritus**

E. H. L. Corwin, Ph.D.,* *Executive Secretary until 1952*
H. D. Kruse, M.D., *Executive Secretary*

* Deceased

Ex Officio

Alexander T. Martin, M.D.
President, The New York Academy of Medicine

Howard Reid Craig, M.D.
Director, The New York Academy of Medicine

SUBCOMMITTEE ON NEONATAL MORTALITY

S. Z. Levine, M.D., *Chairman*

Albert H. Aldridge, M.D.
Harry S. Altman, M.D.
Dorothy H. Andersen, M.D.
Murray H. Bass, M.D.
Eugene S. Coler, M.D.*
Robert L. Craig, M.D.
Joseph Dancis, M.D.
Richard L. Day, M.D.
D. Anthony D'Esopo, M.D.
Adolph G. De Sanctis, M.D.
Samuel W. Dooley, M.D.
R. Gordon Douglas, M.D.
Milton J. Goodfriend, M.D.
Carl T. Javert, M.D.
Alexander T. Martin, M.D.
Harvey B. Matthews, M.D.
John B. Pastore, M.D.*
Oscar M. Schloss, M.D.*
William E. Studdiford, M.D.
Frederick H. Wilke, M.D.

* Deceased

EDITORIAL COMMITTEE

Milton J. Goodfriend, M.D., *Chairman*

Dorothy H. Andersen, M.D.
John W. Fertig, Ph.D.
Richard L. Day, M.D.

FIELD TEAM

Lawrence J. Caruso, M.D.
William F. Finn, M.D.
Martha L. Smith, M.D.
William M. Wiseman, M.D.
Martha Gonski
Alice Gonski

Preface

IN the fall of 1949 a Subcommittee on Neonatal Mortality was appointed by the Committee on Public Health Relations of The New York Academy of Medicine to investigate the perinatal deaths that occurred in New York City in 1950. The Subcommittee consisted of twenty-one members: nine obstetricians, nine pediatricians and three pathologists.[1] The first meeting was held on November 2, 1949 with the then President of the Academy of Medicine, Dr. B. P. Watson, in the chair.

The Subcommittee was instructed to study the causes of perinatal deaths in the city and to determine as accurately as possible the number which with better care might have been prevented. Plans for the study were formulated; funds were secured from a number of foundations. Dr. N. Chandler Foot was appointed Director of the study (March 1, 1950) and Dr. John W. Fertig, Professor of Biostatistics, Columbia University School of Public Health, accepted the post of statistical advisor. Following the selection of a team of field workers[1] and advisory panels of review,[2] the assembling and critical analysis of the data by these two groups progressed

[1] The members of these committees are listed on page vi.

[2] Each advisory panel consisted of one obstetrician, one pediatrician, and one pathologist from the Subcommittee. A number of such reviewing panels served on a rotating basis throughout the period of the collection of the data.

under the able direction of Dr. Foot throughout the remainder of 1950 and well into 1951.

In the fall of 1951 the material was compiled and a draft of the results of the study was prepared by Dr. Foot. This draft was presented to an editorial committee[1] of the Subcommittee for review and editing. In the course of their editorial activities this Committee reached the conclusion that much valuable material which had been obtained in the field and was on file could with advantage be incorporated in the final document for publication. Since Dr. Foot's tenure of office had reached the expiration date of December 1, 1951, according to the terms of his appointment, when this decision was made by the Editorial Committee, the task of incorporating the desired data and revising the manuscript became the responsibility of the Committee.

It soon became evident that such an undertaking would require the services of a full-time person. By a happy coincidence Dr. Schuyler G. Kohl, Associate Professor of Obstetrics and Gynecology, State University of New York College of Medicine at New York City, received a fellowship at this time from the Commonwealth Fund to work in Dr. Fertig's department in the Columbia School of Public Health for his doctorate in public health. This publication is in large part the product of his labors in fulfilling the requirements for his degree. The manuscript was submitted to the Academy for review and revision and it has been approved in its final form by the Committee on Public Health Relations.

This prolonged investigation was made possible by generous grants from five foundations: The Commonwealth Fund, The Association for the Aid of Crippled Children, The Milbank Memorial Fund, The New York Foundation and The New York Fund for Children. During the often slow advance of the study and the occasional vicissitudes through which it passed, none of the contributors lost faith in the undertaking.

To Dr. Foot, Dr. Kohl and Dr. Fertig, to the field team, to the members of the panels, to the Editorial Committee, and to the contributing agencies, the Subcommittee is indebted for their patience and unstinting cooperation.

The Committee would like to acknowledge also the invaluable assistance of Miss Lois Stice in the readying of the manuscript for publication.

The Committee on Public Health Relations of The New York Academy of Medicine is publishing the results of this study in book form with the hope that by illuminating the problem it will contribute to the reduction of perinatal mortality, in the same way as the Committee's earlier publication in 1933 served as a stimulus to the lowering of maternal mortality.

S. Z. LEVINE, M.D.

Foreword

THIS volume contains the report of the second and final phase of an intensive study of infant mortality in New York City, undertaken in 1948 by the Committee on Public Health Relations of The New York Academy of Medicine at the request of the New York City Department of Health, through Dr. Leona Baumgartner, then Chief of the Bureau of Child Hygiene, now Commissioner of Health.

The first part of the study dealt with hospital facilities for infant and maternal care, the report of which was published in 1952 under the title *Infant and Maternal Care in New York City*. A team consisting of an obstetrician and a pediatric nurse, later assisted by a pediatrician, made personal visits to 104 hospitals having maternity services; the hospitals also cooperated by completing a detailed questionnaire. The results of that investigation formed the background for the clinical study of almost 1000 individual infant deaths, herein presented mainly in statistical form.

The procedures used in this study of 955 stillbirths and neonatal deaths in New York City are described in the Introduction; namely, the collection of data, its arrangement and analysis by the staff and review by panels consisting of members of the Subcommittee which carried the project through to the end.

In Chapter I the nature of the data as representative of the perinatal mortality in New York City is examined in many aspects—by weight, age at death, color and sex of the infants, by age and parity of the mothers, by month of death, by place of birth (home or hospital) and borough of birth.

Chapter II sets forth the panel's judgment as to the preventability of the deaths studied and the factors responsible for them, particularly errors in management which may be avoided in the future.

The quality of obstetrical care is subjected to critical analysis in Chapter III. The type of hospital, the number of prenatal visits, the type of professional service given, and the place of death are taken into consideration.

In Chapter IV the author turns to characteristics of the mothers which might have played a part in the deaths of their infants. Such factors include age, number of previous children, past obstetrical history, and the presence or absence of toxemia at delivery.

The next chapter looks into the possible role of analgesia and anesthesia in perinatal mortality.

Chapter VI is devoted to the method of delivery, including a classification of the deaths according to presentation of the infant. The author points out that for a better interpretation of the effects of the method of delivery a study of a sample of all births in the city, not merely of deaths, would be required.

Chapter VII records the time of death of the infants and its relation to preventability.

Perhaps the most important section of the book is Chapter VIII, which deals with the causes of death. In it the author shows how it was necessary to compare and at times to reconcile three sources of information in order to arrive at true causes of death. He discusses in detail the lack of agreement often found among the three sources. He has also analyzed the causes found as they relate to the type of professional service.

Chapter IX summarizes the findings of the study, set forth in twenty-four points. Finally, the author offers a number of suggestions that may be of value to the future investigator in the preparation of similar studies.

MILTON J. GOODFRIEND, M.D.

Acknowledgments

ACKNOWLEDGMENT is made to the following individuals for assistance in making this study possible and aiding in its completion: Doctors Jean A. Curran, Louis M. Hellman, Jacob Yerushalmy, Samuel Z. Levine, Richard L. Day, Dorothy H. Andersen, Milton J. Goodfriend, and Leon Chesley. The following organizations also extended important aid and assistance: The Commonwealth Fund; Columbia University School of Public Health; State University of New York, College of Medicine at New York City; The New York Academy of Medicine; New York City Health Department.

Special acknowledgment is made to Doctor John W. Fertig. Not only has he been a constant advisor and supporter, but he has also generously given innumerable hours in the preparation and editing of the manuscript.

Final thanks are extended to Miss Betsy Aaron for typing the manuscript.

SCHUYLER G. KOHL, M.D.

Contents

Topical List of Tables

PERINATAL MORTALITY IN NEW YORK CITY

INTRODUCTION

Collection and Analysis of the Data

THIS STUDY of perinatal[1] mortality was instituted by The New York Academy of Medicine in 1950. It was planned to cover perinatal mortality for that year in the five boroughs of New York City. The original plan, which included the perinatal mortality of 1950 alone, had to be abandoned because the study could not be started promptly on January 1. It was started in February on a small scale. In order to insure that an entire calendar year was covered and to have the sample reach a predetermined size, it was necessary to extend the study until April 1, 1951.

Certain difficulties arose in the evaluation of the sample as representative of the city as a whole. It was desirable, of course, to compare figures for the same span of time. It was found, however, that 1950 data were not available for every item necessary for comparison; in several instances, therefore, figures for 1949 were used. This interfered with a true comparison because the number of perinatal deaths differed for the two years.

The data were gathered by a staff appointed by the Subcommittee on Neonatal Mortality of the Committee on Public Health Relations of The New York Academy of Medicine.

1 "Perinatal mortality" is a relatively new term which has recently come into wide use. It is an inclusive term covering both stillbirths and neonatal deaths.

PURPOSES

The purposes of the study are:

1. To determine, as accurately as possible, the causes of perinatal mortality.
2. To determine the extent of preventability of perinatal deaths.
3. To supply additional pertinent information concerning perinatal mortality, which cannot be collected by the usual vital statistics records. These additional data include such information as:
   a. Prenatal care
   b. Medical care
   c. Analgesia and anesthesia
   d. Past obstetrical history
   e. Detailed pathologic findings

Vital statistics records as collected and analyzed by local, state, and national health agencies present data from which may be computed detailed stillbirth and neonatal death rates for the entire population. These records also present data on causes of death, color, sex, age, time of death, type of operation for delivery, duration of pregnancy, maternal complications, Rh status, and many similar details. The present study has permitted an evaluation of the accuracy of such information.

METHODS

Photostatic copies of stillbirth and death certificates for infants beyond 28 weeks' gestation or over 1000 grams' birth weight were supplied by the New York City Department of Health. Copies of the matched birth certificates were also supplied. As the stillbirth and death certificates were received, they were classified into categories designated A, B, and C and put up in packets of 100 each.

The categories were as follows:

A Stillbirths
B Neonatal deaths within first five days
C Neonatal deaths from sixth to thirtieth day

The Subcommittee on Neonatal Mortality had decided that the study should include 1000 perinatal deaths and that the composition of the sample should be as follows:

Stillbirths (A)	250 infants
Early neonatal deaths (B)	500
Late neonatal deaths (C)	250

In order to have the desired number of cases in each category, it was necessary to determine what percentage of each category should be sampled. These sampling percentages were set up by examining the reports of the Department of Health for the year 1949.

On the basis of the percentages thus obtained, the proper number of death and stillbirth certificates were selected from each packet of 100; a table of random numbers was used for this purpose. The percentages originally used did not supply the desired number of certificates for each category, and it was therefore necessary to revise the sampling percentages upward. The reasons for this were: (1) the number of perinatal deaths in 1950 was somewhat different from the number in 1949, on which the percentages had been estimated; and (2) some of the certificates were not available for sampling. The details of the sampling percentages and some of the difficulties involved in sampling are discussed in Chapter I.

A special staff of physicians was assigned to complete the obstetrical, pediatric, and pathologic records for each death. The record forms which they used were based upon forms used by the Philadelphia Department of Health in a similar study (Appendix I, Forms 1–3).

It was necessary for the investigators to examine the hospital records of the mother and the infant in order to complete the records for the study. Frequently, further consultation with nurses, house staff, or private physicians was required; although, unfortunately, this was not always accomplished. The nurse member of the investigating staff also made home visits to obtain additional information.

The reports prepared by the investigators were examined by the original Director, who selected for review by the Subcommittee on Neonatal Mortality those which were not clear-cut. These were referred to panels constituted from the Subcommittee. There were several such panels, each consisting of one obstetrician, one pediatrician, and one pathologist. The panels reviewed all the referred cases for preventability, the factors of responsibility, and the causes of death. The investigators were present at the meetings of these panels to supply additional information from their notes. The ultimate results represent the composite judgment of the groups after differences of opinion had been resolved through a full discussion.

At the end of this procedure, all cases had been classified as:

1. Not preventable
2. Preventable
3. Doubtfully preventable
4. Unclassified

The records were further marked as to the presence of one or more of the following responsibility factors (regardless of preventability):

1. Inadequate prenatal care
2. Error in medical judgment
3. Error in medical technique
4. Family at fault
5. Unqualified medical attendant
6. Unavoidable disaster
7. Inadequate pediatric care

The summary sheet (Appendix I, Form 4) was also marked to indicate the cause of death.

Early in 1952, the present author undertook a new study of this mass of data in cooperation with an Editorial Committee consisting of an obstetrician, a pediatrician, a biostatistician, and a pathologist especially qualified in fetal pathology.

There were three types of records: the clinical records of the hospitals, the pathologic reports, and the death certificates. All the material assembled by the original staff was first examined by the author; records on approximately 300 cases were reviewed by the Editorial Committee.

The Editorial Committee considered the clinical record which was on the hospital chart, and if there was a diagnosis other than prematurity on the clinical record, that diagnosis stood; it was never reversed by the Committee. If prematurity was given as the cause of death, the case was then treated as one with no cause listed. In all clinical records where there was no diagnosis or where the diagnosis was expressed as "prematurity," the panel made a clinical diagnosis.

In many of the original investigations the pathologic reports were not complete. In some instances the death certificate indicated that an autopsy had been performed, but there was no report of it; in others, interviews with attending physicians revealed that there had been an autopsy, again without a record in the files of the study. At times the pathologist's report would contain only gross observations without microscopic findings.

In the new study an effort was made to procure the missing data in these cases. The hospitals where delivery was performed or where death occurred were visited; private physicians were consulted. Hospital pathologists prepared reports not previously available for some of the cases; in other instances incomplete or ambiguous reports were completed or clarified by the author or the Editorial Committee. Thus some data not available in 1950 could be incorporated into the study. This supplementary information contributed much to the accuracy of the final determination of the causes of death.

Rarely did the pathologist give a cause of death. Rather, he listed the gross and microscopic observations. On the basis of these and in full knowledge of the clinical diagnosis, the Committee always made the pathologic diagnosis. In not a few cases the pathologic diagnosis was at variance with the clinical diagnosis which the Committee had previously made. This, of course, frequently occurs in actual practice, inasmuch as the pathologic observations shed new light. Of course, prematurity was never given as a pathologic diagnosis.

Prior to coding, the records of each case were independently reviewed by the author and classified as to preventability and the presence of responsibility factors. After this second judgment was rendered, it was compared with that made in the original study. If there was complete agreement, a code sheet (Appendix I, Form 5) was prepared and sent for punching on an 80-column IBM card. When the opinion of the author differed from the original decision as to preventability of a death, the Editorial Committee ruled on the final classification. The Committee's decisions were final.

The death certificate was never changed or reversed for purposes of the study. Usually the physician who submitted the clinical report was not the one who signed the death certificate. Actually, the only reason for bringing the death certificate into the study was to show its relatively great inaccuracy.

In the course of the review, it became necessary to exclude certain cases which had previously been included. These were dropped for the following reasons:

1. Birth weight less than 1000 grams
2. Age at death greater than 30 days
3. Duplication of cases
4. Incomplete records:
   no record for mother
   no pediatric record

After these incomplete records had been rejected there remained in the study fewer than the originally collected 1000 deaths. Following are the numbers of deaths in each category:

Stillbirths (A)	237
Early Neonatal Deaths (B)	483
Late Neonatal Deaths (C)	235
Total	955

An examination of the published reports of the Health Department for 1950 revealed that the numbers of cases in the various categories of the sample bore the following relationships to these categories for New York City:

Category	*Sampling Fraction*	*Weighting Factor*
A	10.2 per cent	6.49
B	28.0 per cent	2.36
C	66.2 per cent	1.00

In considering certain items in the study, it is desirable to speak of the entire perinatal mortality (A + B + C), or the entire neonatal mortality (B + C). Before the addition can be performed, it is necessary to weight the categories in accordance with the sampling fractions involved. For example, whereas the A's represent one-half of the city's perinatal mortality, they represent only one-fourth of the study. The appropriate weighting factors, which are based on the sampling ratios, are noted above. When appropriately weighted, the sample of 955 deaths represents a cross section of the perinatal mortality (A + B + C) of the city for 1950.

It was not the purpose of this study to duplicate information available from vital statistics records, but rather to concentrate on preventability, responsibility, causes of death, and related clinical data. The stillbirth rate and neonatal death rates were available for the entire 1950 experience. It was not necessary to secure a sample to supply these data, but such items as prenatal care, toxemia, preventability, analgesia, anesthesia, type of medical attendant, evaluation of pediatric care, and the like were either not obtainable for the entire city experience, or were not reliably reported. It was this type of information, in addition to responsibility factors and causes of death, which was sought in this analysis.

All data in this study relate to deaths, and there is no comparable information available for the surviving infants. This lack prevents a highly desirable type of comparison. Corresponding information for surviving infants (or all infants) would require a sample of all births. With the data here presented, the importance of the clinical items noted as relevant factors in perinatal mortality cannot be evaluated; nor do they necessarily reflect the frequency of these factors in the total number of births.

Throughout the analysis the records of the premature and the mature infants are treated separately. For the purposes of this study a premature infant was defined as one weighing more than 1000 grams but less than 2500 grams. By definition, all infants above 2500 grams are considered mature.

The study includes 477 premature infants as follows:

A (Stillbirths)	110
B (Early neonatal deaths)	279
C (Late neonatal deaths)	88

There were also 478 mature infants as follows:

A (Stillbirths)	127
B (Early neonatal deaths)	204
C (Late neonatal deaths)	147

CHAPTER I

Evaluation of the Sample

In order to make clear the framework of this study of perinatal deaths, it is necessary to explain the extent to which the sample represented the whole experience of New York City in 1950. In point of time, the sample was not strictly representative, in that 187 cases were drawn from deaths that occurred in the first quarter of 1951. As was stated in the Introduction, all the death certificates routed to the study were sampled at random. However, not all of the certificates were available for sampling. After the 1950 data for the city became available, comparisons were made for certain pertinent items; in some instances the information was not available for 1950, and it was necessary to use figures for 1949. The tables that follow in this chapter indicate the year for which the comparison was made.

SIZE OF SAMPLE

The sampling percentages originally contemplated for the A, B, and C categories were set as shown in Table I. An analysis of the data for the perinatal deaths in the city in 1949 had indicated that these percentages would give the desired 250 A, 500 B and 250 C cases.

The number of perinatal deaths available for sampling in 1950 was somewhat different, however, from the number

Table I. Proposed Sampling Percentages

A	B	C
10	25	50

Table II. Working Sampling Percentages

A	B	C
17	35	80

in the city experience of 1949. This difference, together with the fact that not all the certificates were available for sampling, necessitated an upward revision in the sampling percentages. Table II sets forth the revision.

On the basis of the data for the city experience of 1950, which later became available, the stillbirths and neonatal deaths actually entering the study constituted the percentages of the 1950 figures which are shown in Table III. The only marked deviation from the originally postulated percentages occurred in the C category. In spite of the agreement, it does not follow that the distribution of the sample was representative of the entire city in all characteristics.

Because the sampling percentages varied from category to category, no analysis of the combined group of perinatal deaths could be made without weighting each group by its appropriate factor. The necessary weighting factors based upon the sampling percentages shown in Table III appear in the third line of the table.

Table III. Actual Sampling Percentages

	A	B	C
Sampling percentage	10.2	28.0	66.2
No. of cases	237	483	235
Weighting coefficient	6.49	2.36	1.00

COMPARISON WITH CITY DATA

Several difficulties arose in a comparison of the sample with the city experience. Occasionally there were discrepancies in birth weights as recorded on the certificate and in the clinical record. The statement on the clinical record was taken to be correct. If it showed a birth weight of 1000 grams or less, the case was eliminated from the study even if the birth weight recorded on the certificate was over 1000 grams. Still other cases were dropped because the clinical records were incomplete. Deaths of infants whose weight was over 1000 grams at birth but incorrectly listed on the death certificates as 1000 grams or under are not represented at all. Essentially, the cases studied constitute a sample of that portion of the city experience of 1950 and the first quarter of 1951, in which the death certificates correctly listed a birth weight of over 1000 grams and in which the clinical records were adequate. An additional difficulty was introduced by the fact that in the case of the stillbirths the city data refer to infants of over 28 weeks' gestation but for neonatal deaths include all infant deaths.

Tables IV and V show the distribution of the stillbirths and neonatal deaths by borough of birth. Table IV demonstrates that the sample is significantly[1] overloaded with

[1] Since the sample formed an appreciable proportion (10.2 per cent) of the stillbirths of the city, this fact must be considered in evaluating the standard error. Thus in the case of Manhattan the standard error appropriate to comparing 34.6 per cent with 25.2 per cent is:

$$\text{S.E.} = \sqrt{\frac{(25.2)\,(100 - 25.2)}{237}} \times \sqrt{1 - .108} = 2.66 \text{ per cent}$$

The difference between 34.6 per cent and 25.2 per cent is equal to 3.46 standard error; this is significant.

The basic data from which the tables in this book have been compiled are on file at The New York Academy of Medicine, where they may be consulted.

Table IV. Percentage Distribution by Borough of Birth—*Stillbirths*

Borough	*Study*	*City 1950*
Manhattan	34.6	25.2
Bronx	14.8	14.7
Brooklyn	29.2	36.4
Queens	16.3	15.4
Richmond	1.3	2.3
Non-resident	3.8	6.0
No. of deaths	*237*	

Table V. Percentage Distribution by Borough of Birth—*Neonatal Deaths*

Borough	*Study, Adjusted*	*City 1950*
Manhattan	31.6	27.2
Bronx	14.5	14.7
Brooklyn	31.9	33.8
Queens	15.7	16.3
Richmond	1.7	2.2
Non-resident	4.6	5.8
No. of deaths	*718*	

Manhattan stillbirths and correspondingly deficient for Brooklyn. The neonatal deaths in the sample are more representative of the city distribution than are the stillbirths. Although there is some "loading" in Manhattan for the neonatal deaths, it attains only borderline significance.

Table VI shows the distribution of the deaths by sex. It is

Table VI. Percentage Distribution of Perinatal Deaths—*By Sex of Infant*

	Stillbirths		*Neonatal Deaths*	
Sex	Study	City 1949	Study, Adjusted	City 1949*
Male	54.7	53.9	61.3	58.0
Female	45.3	46.1	38.7	42.0
No. of deaths	*237*		*718*	

* 1950 data not obtainable.

Table VII. Percentage Distribution of Perinatal Deaths—*By Color*

	Stillbirths		Neonatal Deaths	
Color	Study	City 1950	Study, Adjusted	City 1950
White	84.0	81.6	83.1	76.9
Non-white	16.0	18.4	16.9	23.1
No. of deaths	*237*		*718*	

readily apparent that for both the stillbirths and neonatal deaths, the agreement between the data in the study and the New York City data for 1949 is satisfactory as to distribution between the sexes.

Table VII shows the distribution of the deaths by color. The distribution of stillbirths is in good agreement with that for the city. The distribution of the neonatal deaths by color, on the other hand, is not in harmony[2] with that for the city.

Table VIII gives the distribution of stillbirths and neonatal deaths by month of occurrence. The sampling of the neonatal deaths by month of occurrence seems to be satisfactory.[3] The sampling of the stillbirths, however, is very poor. This is related to the difficulties resulting from irregu-

[2] To test whether the figure 83.1 per cent of white among the neonatal deaths of the sample is significantly different from the 76.9 per cent for the city (Table VII), it is necessary to correct for the fact that the sample forms an appreciable proportion of the city experience, and also for the fact that the early (B) and late (C) neonatal deaths do not form the same sampling proportion. Assuming that the percentage of white (in the city) does not differ greatly for the B's and C's, the appropriate standard error may be written as follows:

$$\text{S.E.} = \sqrt{\frac{76.9 \times 23.1\,[3.57\,(3.57 - 1)\,483 + 1.51\,(1.51 - 1)\,235]}{[(3.57 \times 483) + (1.51 \times 235)]^2}}$$

$$\text{S.E.} = 1.52 \text{ per cent}$$

3.57 and 1.51 are the reciprocals of the sampling proportion for B and C, respectively, and 483 and 235 are the respective totals for B and C. The difference, 6.2 per cent, is significant, since it is equal to 4.07 standard error.

[3] Chi square with 11 degrees of freedom, uncorrected for stratification and the sampling percentage, is 182 for the neonatal deaths. This is not statistically significant.

Table VIII. Percentage Distribution of Perinatal Deaths—
By Month of Death

	Stillbirths		*Neonatal Deaths*	
Month	Study	City 1950	Study, Adjusted	City 1949*
January	10.5	8.4	9.2	7.6
February	12.2	7.9	7.8	7.4
March	14.8	9.6	6.0	8.5
April	6.3	8.2	7.5	7.9
May	13.5	8.6	9.0	8.8
June	2.5	7.7	8.2	8.4
July	3.8	7.9	8.3	8.9
August	7.2	7.3	8.2	9.0
September	8.4	8.0	7.6	9.1
October	7.2	9.1	9.2	7.4
November	4.2	8.8	9.0	8.7
December	9.4	8.5	10.0	8.3
No. of deaths	*237*		*718*	

* 1950 data not available.

larity of submission of certificates and from the fact that 28 per cent of the stillbirths were drawn from the first quarter of 1951, while only 9 per cent of the neonatal deaths were drawn from the first quarter of 1951.

Tables IX and X show that for both the stillbirths and the neonatal deaths, the sample agrees satisfactorily in respect to birth weight and to age of the mother.

Table IX. Percentage Distribution of Perinatal Deaths—*By Birth Weight*

	Stillbirths		*Neonatal Deaths*	
Weight (grams)	Study	City 1950	Study, Adjusted	City 1949*
1001–1499	10.1	12.9	19.1	18.2
1500–1999	11.2	15.5	19.3	17.1
2000–2499	11.2	16.0	15.8	15.1
2500–2999	19.7	17.2	19.1	17.9
3000–3499	19.7	17.5	15.8	18.5
3500–3999	15.4	12.5	7.3	9.2
4000–4499	6.9	4.7	2.7	3.1
4500–4999	2.1	2.1	0.5	0.7
5000 and over	3.7	1.6	0.4	0.2
No. of deaths	*188*		*718*	

* 1950 data not obtainable.

Table X. Percentage Distribution of Perinatal Deaths—*By Age of Mother*

	Stillbirths		*Neonatal Deaths*	
Age of Mother	Study	City 1950	Study, Adjusted	City 1950
Under 15	0.0	0.2	0.2	0.1
15–19	3.8	5.5	7.2	7.7
20–24	23.2	23.6	26.5	27.8
25–29	28.3	29.2	29.9	29.6
30–34	23.6	23.0	19.6	19.4
35–39	17.3	14.4	11.8	12.8
40–44	3.8	3.8	4.3	2.3
45–49	0.0	0.2	0.4	0.3
50 and over	0.0	0.0	0.1	0.0
No. of deaths	*237*		*718*	

Table XI. Percentage Distribution of Perinatal Deaths—*By Place of Birth*

	Stillbirths		*Neonatal Deaths*	
Place of Birth	Study	City 1949*	Study, Adjusted	City 1949*
Voluntary hospital	56.1	55.7	55.3	58.1
Government hospital	21.5	21.8	23.6	27.6
Proprietary hospital	21.9	18.4	17.9	12.6
Home delivery	0.5	4.1	3.2	1.7
No. of deaths	*237*		*718*	

* 1950 data not obtainable.

Table XII. Percentage Distribution by Parity of Mother—*Stillbirths*

Parity	*Study*	*City 1949**
1st child	38.4	38.7
2nd child	27.4	23.0
3rd child	12.7	15.4
4th child	8.4	9.2
5th child	3.8	4.5
6th child	1.3	2.4
7th child	0.8	1.8
8th child	0.8	0.9
9th child	1.7	0.5
10th child or more	1.7	1.8
Unknown parity	3.0	1.8
No. of deaths	*237*	

* 1950 data not obtainable.

Table XI shows the distribution of the perinatal deaths by place of birth. The study's data on stillbirths agree quite well with those of the city, except for home deliveries. The sample included only 1 stillbirth at home instead of the expected 10. In spite of the slight discrepancies in the case of the neonatal deaths, the agreement may be considered satisfactory.

Table XII shows satisfactory agreement between the sample and the city in respect to parity of mother for the stillbirths. Corresponding information was not obtainable for the neonatal deaths.

Table XIII gives the distribution of neonatal deaths by age at death. In further testing the study data to ascertain their suitability as a representative sample of the city, a dissimilarity was found concerning the age of neonatal death. The lack of agreement may be due to the fact that the deaths in the sample were selected on the basis of birth weight, whereas the figures for the entire city refer to infants of 28 or more weeks' gestation, regardless of birth weight.

In spite of the difficulties of sampling and the differences in criteria, the sample may be considered satisfactory.

Table XIII. Percentage Distribution of Neonatal Deaths—
By Age at Death

Age at Death	*Study, Adjusted*	*City 1950*
First 24 hours	46.5	42.0
24–48 hours	20.5	16.8
48 hours–5 days	15.8	24.1
6 days–30 days	17.2	17.1
No. of deaths	*718*	

CHAPTER II

Preventability and Responsibility

THIS chapter reports the evaluation of the management of the cases in terms of preventability of and circumstantial responsibility for death. An attempt was made to record errors in management, to classify them, and to assess the preventability of the death. The method of evaluation was described in the Introduction.

Table XIV indicates the percentage of deaths in each category, for mature and premature infants, which was deemed by the Committee to be preventable.[1] It also gives

Table XIV. Frequency of Preventability of Death* (Per Cent)—
For 955 Perinatal Deaths

	A	*B*	*C*	*Adjusted Total†* *(A+B+C)*
Premature	23	32	52	29
Mature	35	53	45	42
All deaths	29	41	48	35

* The terms "frequency of preventability," "preventability frequency," "preventability rate," and sometimes "preventability," are used interchangeably throughout the presentation. The terms refer to the percentages of the deaths that were deemed preventable.

† The figure of 29 per cent for deaths of premature infants was obtained by using the weighting coefficients, given in the Introduction, as follows:

$$\frac{(25 \times 6.49) + (90 \times 2.36) + (46 \times 1.0)}{(110 \times 6.49) + (279 \times 2.36) + (88 \times 1.0)} = 28.8 \text{ per cent}$$

The numbers in the numerator (25, 90, and 46) represent the preventable deaths of premature infants in categories A, B, and C, respectively. The numbers in the denominator (110, 279, and 88) represent the deaths of premature infants in each category.

[1] Preventable, doubtfully preventable, and unclassified.

the percentage of preventability for each category and for premature and mature infants separately.

In the A and B categories, the percentages of the deaths which were preventable are greater for the mature infants than for the premature ones. Generally the preventability increases from category A to category C. It is important to note that deaths adjudged preventable are 1.45 times as frequent in the mature infants as in the premature. It is among mature infants that the obstetrician and pediatrician have the greatest opportunity to save lives.

RESPONSIBILITY FACTORS

Responsibility factors were classified into eight groups, as follows:

Inadequate prenatal care
Errors in medical judgment
Errors in medical technique
Unqualified medical attendant
Family at fault
Intercurrent infection
Unavoidable disaster
Unsatisfactory pediatric care

Following are case summaries that illustrate one or more of these factors.

Inadequate prenatal care

1. A 20-year-old unmarried woman made her first and only prenatal visit during the sixth month of gestation. She was not seen again by a physician until the onset of labor. One-half hour prior to the delivery of the first of triplets, she was seen by her family physician. She was delivered of the three infants at home. The smallest weighed 1216 grams. All three succumbed in the neonatal period. The third is the

only one included in this study. The death was classified as non-preventable, and the chief responsibility factor was "unavoidable disaster." The other responsibility factors present were: inadequate prenatal care and family at fault.

2. A 28-year-old para 0–0–0–0[2] who had been a known diabetic for nineteen years had received more or less regular prenatal care. In spite of this attention, she had suffered attacks of kidney infection with acidosis on two occasions. She was admitted to the hospital at term in diabetic acidosis and shock and in labor. After fourteen hours of labor she was delivered by cesarean section of an infant weighing 3430 grams. The child was in poor condition at birth, and developed an infection which was not recognized for four days. He died in spite of intensive therapy. This death was deemed preventable on the basis of three factors: inadequate prenatal care, error in medical judgment, and unsatisfactory pediatric care.

Errors in medical judgment

A 46-year-old woman, para 8–0–0–8, was admitted to the hospital seven hours after the membranes had been ruptured artificially in order to induce labor. Since labor did not ensue, induction was attempted by the introduction of a No. 4 hydrostatic bag. When this also failed to initiate contractions, the patient was given pituitary stimulation. Shortly thereafter she precipitously delivered an infant weighing 4850 grams. The infant was in poor condition; it showed signs typical of intracranial hemorrhage and subsequently succumbed to this condition. It was an error in medical judgment to administer pituitrin to a woman of advanced age and advanced parity. This death was judged to have been preventable.

[2] The code used in these case reports is as follows: the first figure is the number of full-term pregnancies; the second, the number of premature births; the third, the number of abortions; the fourth, the number of living children.

Errors in medical technique

A 30-year-old patient who had previously had one full-term delivery had received adequate prenatal care and was admitted to the hospital at term in active labor with a frank breech presentation. The first and second stages of labor covered eleven and one-half hours. After thirty minutes of second stage it was elected to deliver the patient by bringing down the feet and performing a breech extraction. The fetal heart tones were of good quality at the onset of the procedure. The delivery was effected without difficulty until attempts were made to deliver the head. It was then necessary to try both Piper and Kjelland forceps. In addition, extreme suprafundic pressure was necessary in order to effect delivery. During this procedure the fetal heart tones were lost. The weight of the infant was not recorded on the chart nor on the stillbirth certificate. The patient was delivered by a junior member of the house staff. This death was deemed to have been preventable. The following responsibility factors were involved: error in medical judgment (improper evaluation of the pelvis prior to delivery in a breech presentation); error in medical technique; and unqualified medical attendant (difficult obstetrical procedure in hands of an inadequately trained obstetrician).

Unqualified medical attendant

A 30-year-old woman had been delivered of a living infant at term and a stillborn infant at term, and had had an abortion of a three months' gestation. The stillbirth occurred after a labor with a breech presentation. The patient was admitted to the hospital in labor. The first and second stages progressed normally. When the cervix was fully dilated and the presenting part was at plus one station, the patient was taken to the delivery room. Suprafundic pressure and "bearing down" by the patient produced no further descent. The fetal heart rate was recorded at 80 beats per minute between uterine contractions.

It was elected to deliver the patient at this time. The position was thought to be left occiput anterior. A mid-pelvic application of axis traction forceps was effected; strong traction produced no descent. It was then noted that the position was right occiput posterior. The fetal heart rate remained depressed.

The physician in charge, who was not a qualified obstetrician, belatedly sought consultation. The consultant applied Kjelland forceps and attempted to rotate the fetal head. This was unsuccessful. Rotation was accomplished manually to left occiput anterior, and Elliott forceps were applied. Strong traction produced no further descent. Suddenly there appeared an excessive amount of bleeding from the uterine cavity. Examination revealed signs typical of rupture of the lower uterine segment. The patient was transferred to the operating room, and her abdomen was opened. There was a transverse rent in the lower uterine segment. Part of the infant protruded through the tear. A supravaginal hysterectomy was performed after a stillborn infant had been delivered. The infant weighed 4500 grams.

This stillbirth was classified as preventable. The responsibility factors were: error in medical judgment; error in medical technique; unqualified medical attendant.

Family at fault

A case in which the family was at fault is described in the following notes by the nurse who visited a home to investigate the death of a 26-day-old baby: "Family lived in small furnished room with poor facilities for caring for baby. Mother worked hard and was careful to see that baby was well cared for. On August 19, 1950, the mother had the baby in bed with her for the 6:30 A.M. feeding. While the baby was nursing, the mother fell asleep. When she awoke one hour later, she was lying on the baby." This death was classified as preventable.

Intercurrent infection

In this case the antepartum course and the delivery were uneventful. The baby had a slight upper respiratory infection when discharged from the hospital—against advice. The parents signed a release August 25, 1950, the third postpartum day. The baby was visited at home that day by the family physician; no therapy was prescribed. The nurse's report of her home visit states: "Mother called M.D. several times but he refused to visit. Baby was constipated, so D.M. #3 was added to the formula. Baby vomited on evening of September 9, but seemed all right. Took 2 A.M. feeding well. When father looked at baby at 3:00 A.M. baby was dead." The police report states: "Baby fed at 2:45 A.M. Mother and father awoke about noon. They found baby dead in crib, on his face." The Medical Examiner's report of death gave the cause as "Bronchopneumonia." This death was classified as preventable, and the responsibility factors were listed as: intercurrent infection, inadequate pediatric care, and family at fault.

Unavoidable disaster

A patient was delivered by breech extraction of a stillborn infant weighing 3884 grams. The fetal heartbeat had disappeared just prior to the delivery, which had occurred after three hours of the second stage of labor, with the breech visible. Autopsy revealed (1) a trilocular heart (one atrium), and (2) transposition of the great vessels. The responsibility factors were: errors in medical judgment; unavoidable disaster.

Unsatisfactory pediatric care

Unsatisfactory pediatric care was amply illustrated in several of the preceding case summaries.

FINDINGS

Table XV demonstrates the frequency of the various responsibility factors in each category for premature and ma-

Table XV. Frequency of Responsibility Factors (Per Cent)—
For 955 Perinatal Deaths

477 PREMATURE INFANTS

Factor	*A*	*B*	*C*	*Adjusted Total*
Inadequate prenatal care	27	18	23	23
Errors in medical judgment	22	34	28	28
Errors in medical technique	5	25	39	16
Unqualified medical attendant	6	4	2	5
Family at fault	4	6	9	5
Intercurrent infection	—	1	13	3
Unavoidable disaster	72	54	33	62
Unsatisfactory pediatric care	—	17	49	21
No. of deaths	*110*	*279*	*88*	

478 MATURE INFANTS

Factor	*A*	*B*	*C*	*Adjusted Total*
Inadequate prenatal care	21	20	12	20
Errors in medical judgment	31	40	32	34
Errors in medical technique	25	46	24	32
Unqualified medical attendant	6	15	3	9
Family at fault	4	2	17	4
Intercurrent infection	—	2	17	5
Unavoidable disaster	57	38	38	49
Unsatisfactory pediatric care	—	31	36	33
No. of deaths	*127*	*204*	*147*	

ture infants, respectively. Since more than one responsibility factor may be present in any given case, the percentages in any category will add to more than 100. The number of perinatal deaths upon which each table is based is recorded on the last line.

The frequency of these responsibility factors in all births in the city is not known. The figures presented here are for deaths only; they do not necessarily reflect the frequency of these factors in the total number of births.

The determination of preventability from a review of records cannot be exact in all instances. It is apparent in the decisions by the panels that individual differences of opinion were constantly at play. These differences were no doubt largely resolved in discussion, but occasional inconsistencies did appear. This is the situation with a death in the B category which was termed "unavoidable disaster" and at the same time deemed preventable. The infant in this case presented a congenital anomaly of the gastrointestinal tract, which was thought to have been amenable to surgery. The early diagnosis essential for proper therapy was not made, and the child died. Hence this case involves two responsibility factors: (1) the anomaly, and (2) the error in medical judgment. An argument so engendered might wax and wane for hours, but the panel had to fix responsibility. The panel's problem was further complicated by the fact that postmortem examinations had been made in only 413 of the deaths.

The task of deciding preventability is often difficult. There is an implication that the child should not have succumbed. The panel could only decide whether or not there was mishandling of the case or that the patient did or did not receive optimal care.

Table XVI. Frequency of Preventability of Death (Per Cent)—
By Responsibility Factors

477 PREMATURE INFANTS

Factors	*A*	*B*	*C*	*Adjusted Total*
PRENATAL CARE				
Adequate	14	27	50	22
Inadequate	47	59	60	52
MEDICAL JUDGMENT				
No errors	6	16	22	12
Errors present	83	64	72	72
MEDICAL TECHNIQUE				
No errors	19	18	26	19
Errors present	100*	73	94	80
MEDICAL ATTENDANT				
Qualified	19	30	51	23
Unqualified	83*	83*	100*	84
FAMILY AT FAULT				
No fault	21	31	49	26
At fault	75*	71*	86*	74
INTERCURRENT INFECTION				
Absent	—	31	55	35
Present	—	25*	36*	30*
UNAVOIDABLE DISASTER				
Present	0	1	0	0.2
Absent	81	70	85	75
PEDIATRIC CARE				
Satisfactory	—	25	20	25
Unsatisfactory	—	66	86	72
All deaths†	23	32	52	29

* Based on less than 20 deaths.
† See Table XIV.

Table XVI shows how the frequency of preventability varies according to the presence or absence of various responsibility factors. The association shown might have been anticipated; that is, the frequency of preventability is greatest where unfavorable responsibility factors are present.

Table XVII shows the frequency of autopsies for each category according to maturity. Table XVIII records the frequency of preventability for each category according to maturity and whether or not an autopsy was performed. It may be noted in Table XVII that the frequency of autopsies

Table XVI (*continued*)

478 MATURE INFANTS

Factors	A	B	C	*Adjusted Total*
PRENATAL CARE				
Adequate	29	48	44	37
Inadequate	56	73	53*	61
MEDICAL JUDGMENT				
No errors	15	32	27	21
Errors present	80	84	83	82
MEDICAL TECHNIQUE				
No errors	19	28	33	23
Errors present	81	81	83	81
MEDICAL ATTENDANT				
Qualified	31	47	44	37
Unqualified	88*	87	75*	87
FAMILY AT FAULT				
No fault	35	52	37	41
At fault	40*	100*	87	66
INTERCURRENT INFECTION				
Absent	—	53	48	52
Present	—	33*	26	27
UNAVOIDABLE DISASTER				
Present	1	0	5	1
Absent	78	84	69	80
PEDIATRIC CARE				
Satisfactory	—	39	23	35
Unsatisfactory	—	83	83	83
All deaths†	35	53	45	42

* Based on less than 20 deaths.
† See Table XIV.

increased from 24 per cent in category A to 54 per cent in category C. The frequency of preventability also increased from category A to category C, as seen in Table XVIII.

This parallelism, which is particularly marked in the case

Table XVII. Frequency of Autopsies (Per Cent)—
For 955 Perinatal Deaths

	A	B	C	*Adjusted Total*
Premature	17	44	52	31
Mature	29	53	54	40
All deaths	24	47	54	35

Table XVIII. Frequency of Preventability of Death (Per Cent)—
By Performance of Autopsy

	A		*B*		*C*		
	Pre-mature	Mature	Pre-mature	Mature	Pre-mature	Mature	*Adjusted Total*
Autopsy	21	38	37	43	50	41	37
No autopsy	23	33	29	64	55	49	34
All deaths*	23	35	32	53	52	45	35

* See Table XIV.

of the premature infants, might at first thought suggest that the performance of autopsies influenced the panel to label a death "preventable." Whether or not an autopsy was performed, however, the frequency of preventability varied but little with maturity status. In only one group, the B mature infants, is the frequency of preventability significantly different for autopsied and non-autopsied infants.

The conclusion is therefore drawn that whether or not an autopsy was performed exerted little or no influence in the determination of preventability.

The following conclusions may be drawn from a study of Tables XV and XVI and the illustrative examples:

1. There was no significant[3] difference in frequencies of inadequate prenatal care among the categories. This is true for both the premature and the mature infants.
2. Errors in medical judgment were somewhat more frequent among the neonatal deaths than among the stillbirths. This was true for both premature and mature infants and is of borderline[4] significance statistically.
3. Errors in medical technique were significantly more frequent in the neonatal deaths than in the stillbirths.

[3] A probability of less than 1 per cent is taken as the criterion of statistical significance.

[4] A probability of between 1 and 5 per cent.

4. "Unqualified medical attendant" was of equal frequency in all categories of premature infants. In the case of mature infants the presence of an unqualified medical attendant was considerably more frequent in the B category than in either A or C categories.
5. "Family at fault" appears to increase from category A through C. This difference is not of statistical significance for the premature infants. In the mature infants, on the other hand, this factor was significantly more frequent in category C. Perhaps this reflects improper care of the infants following discharge from the hospital. Inasmuch as a mature infant is more likely to be released from the hospital and to contract a fatal disease at home than is the premature infant, this finding is not surprising.
6. Intercurrent infection was significantly more frequent in the C category than in the B category. This is true for both premature and mature infants. Intercurrent infection was most frequently the responsibility factor present in the cases of infants who had been discharged from the hospital.
7. Unavoidable disaster is of greatest frequency in the stillbirths. This is true for both the premature and the mature infants.
8. Unsatisfactory pediatric care is significantly more frequent in the C category than in the B group of premature infants. The difference for the mature infants is not significant.

CHAPTER III

Obstetrical Care

IN THE recent past great strides have been made in obstetrical care. The development of prenatal care and the elaboration of new obstetrical techniques, along with advances in care of the newborn, are thought to be largely responsible for the continuing decrease in perinatal mortality rates. It is therefore important that the relationships between obstetrical care and perinatal mortality be explored. This chapter deals with some of those relationships.

TYPE OF HOSPITAL SERVICE

Table XIX shows the distribution of the perinatal deaths in the study according to the type of hospital care and the maturity status. It may be seen from this table that the relationship of prematurity to maturity was 1 to 1 in both private and ward cases. Moreover, there was no deviation from this ratio among the categories.

Table XIX. Percentage Distribution of Deaths—*By Type of Hospital Care and Maturity Status*

Degree of Maturity	*A*		*B*		*C*		*Adjusted Total*	
	Private	Ward	Private	Ward	Private	Ward	Private	Ward
Premature	65	35	56	44	55	45	60	40
Mature	57	43	66	34	55	45	59	41
All degrees	61	39	61	39	55	45	59	41

Table XX. Frequency of Preventability of Death (Per Cent)—
By Service Status

PREMATURE INFANTS

	A	B	C	Adjusted Total
Private	21	30	44	26
Ward	26	36	63	33
All deaths*	23	32	52	29

* See Table XIV.

MATURE INFANTS

	A	B	C	Adjusted Total
Private	29	49	45	38
Ward	42	59	46	47
All deaths*	35	53	45	42

* See Table XIV.

The proportion of private care in the study, 59 per cent of the perinatal deaths, is comparable with that of the city-wide experience for the year 1949. In that year the percentage of private care for all infants who were stillborn or who died in the neonatal period was 57. In regard to type of hospital care, it appears that the survey is representative. These percentages apply, not to all births, but only to stillbirths and neonatal deaths.

Table XX presents the frequency of preventability by type of hospital care for the deaths of premature and mature infants, respectively. The data reveal that throughout all categories and in each maturity status a greater proportion of the deaths on ward service than of deaths on private service was classified as preventable. This may indicate that, in the judgment of the panels, preventable deaths were less likely to occur among private patients than among ward service patients. This matter will be discussed at greater length in the section concerned with specific types of hospitals.

Table XXI. Percentage Distribution of Perinatal Deaths—
By Number of Prenatal Visits

	Adjusted Total	
No. of Visits	Premature	Mature
None	13	8
1–3	12	9
4–8	20	24
9 or more	11	22
Unknown	44	37
Total	100	100

PRENATAL CARE

Table XXI demonstrates the distribution of deaths of premature and mature infants according to the number of prenatal visits. It is clearly seen that information regarding this item was not completely collected in the survey. In 44 per cent of the case records there was no mention of the number of prenatal visits. With such a large proportion of the records in the "unknown" group, it is advisable not to draw conclusions, but only to note the incompleteness of the information. It may be of importance to state that practically all of the records that were incomplete in this respect were those of private patients. In any event, these data pertain only to deaths and give no information on all births.

Table XXII gives the frequency of preventability accord-

Table XXII. Frequency of Preventability of Death (Per Cent)—
By Number of Prenatal Visits

	Adjusted Total	
No. of Visits	Premature	Mature
None	37	43
1–3	27	44
4–8	30	51
9 or more	39	34
Unknown	23	40
All deaths	29	42

ing to the number of prenatal visits. If the records had been sufficiently informative in regard to number of prenatal visits, it would have been of interest to compare preventability in this chart with inadequate prenatal care as described in the preceding chapter.

TYPE OF PROFESSIONAL SERVICE

Table XXIII records the percentage distribution of deaths in premature and mature infants, respectively, according to the type of professional service.

Table XXIV shows the frequency of preventability for deaths of premature and mature infants according to the type of professional service. Examination of the adjusted total for each specified type of professional service reveals that for both the premature and the mature infants, the house staff has the highest frequency associated with deaths characterized as preventable. For the premature infants, the second highest rate of preventable deaths is recorded for the obstetricians, while for the mature infant deaths, the second highest is recorded for the "other physicians."

Closer scrutiny reveals that (1) "other physicians" are associated with the highest frequency of preventable deaths in three of the categories and in a fourth are tied with the house

Table XXIII. Percentage Distribution of Perinatal Deaths—
By Type of Professional Service

	Adjusted Total	
Type of Service	Premature	Mature
House staff	25	32
Obstetricians	19	22
Other physicians	42	37
Unknown care	14	9
Total	100	100

Table XXIV. Frequency of Preventability of Death (Per Cent)—
By Type of Professional Service

PREMATURE INFANTS

Type of Service	A	B	C	*Adjusted Total*
House staff	30	32	54	32
Obstetricians	33*	26	31	29
Other physicians	18	32	59	25
Unknown care	17*	41	75*	36
All deaths†	23	32	52	29

* Based on less than 20 deaths.
† See Table XIV.

MATURE INFANTS

Type of Service	A	B	C	*Adjusted Total*
House staff	47	53	46	48
Obstetricians	30	33	37	32
Other physicians	29	57	48	42
Unknown care	11*	70	45*	30
All deaths†	35	53	45	42

* Based on less than 20 deaths.
† See Table XIV.

staff, (2) the house staff is the highest in only one of the categories but is tied with "other physicians" in one additional category, and (3) the obstetricians are associated with the highest frequency of deaths characterized as preventable in only one of the six categories, premature stillbirths. This category, premature stillborn infants, includes only 15 deaths, however, and thus the higher value for the obstetricians may be due to chance. It should be noted that because of the high weighting coefficient for stillbirths, 6.49, the adjusted total is greatly affected by the preventability rates among the stillbirths.

The results of these comparisons are not surprising. It might have been anticipated that patients cared for by obstetricians would contribute the fewest preventable deaths. On the other hand, many patients cared for by the house staff had had no prenatal attention, and the preventability "rate"

Table XXV. Frequency of Responsibility Factors (Per Cent)—
By Type of Professional Service

PREMATURE INFANTS

	Adjusted Totals		
Responsibility Factors	House Staff	Obstetricians	Other Physicians
Inadequate prenatal care	32	7*	11*
Error in medical judgment	32	33	27
Error in medical technique	16	17	17
Unqualified medical attendant	3*	—	9*
Intercurrent infection	2*	2*	1*
Family at fault	5*	1*	2*
Unavoidable disaster	59	63	66
Unsatisfactory pediatric care	16*	14*	27
No. of deaths	*123*	*107*	*170*

* Based on less than 20 deaths.

MATURE INFANTS

	Adjusted Totals		
Responsibility Factors	House Staff	Obstetricians	Other Physicians
Inadequate prenatal care	27	10*	11
Error in medical judgment	56	27	37
Error in medical technique	35	18	36
Unqualified medical attendant	3*	1*	18
Intercurrent infection	2*	1*	2*
Family at fault	8	—	2*
Unavoidable disaster	40	62	49
Unsatisfactory pediatric care	28	22*	40
No. of deaths	*130*	*102*	*185*

* Based on less than 20 deaths.

for them need not really reflect any lack of skill on the part of the house staff.

Table XXV gives the frequency of responsibility factors for each type of professional service. In the delivery of mature infants who did not survive, the house staff frequently committed errors in medical judgment. In any event these errors account in part for the relatively lower frequency of preventability in cases attended by obstetricians and other physicians. It will be recalled that this responsibility factor is associated with a high preventability rate.

Among the deaths of premature infants, errors in medical

technique were committed with equal frequency by all three categories of doctors. On the other hand, in the management of the delivery of mature infants resulting in death, errors were made with equal frequency by the house staff and other physicians, but only about one-half as frequently by the obstetrician group. This lower frequency of errors in technique results in a decreased frequency of preventability for the obstetrician group.

There are no significant differences in the occurrence of intercurrent infection among the various groups and maturity states.

"Unqualified medical attendant" accrues to the disadvantage of the "other physicians." This factor is highest for the "other physicians," quite low for the house staff and practically non-existent for the obstetricians. It also carries a high frequency of preventability.

Without question, the responsibility factor, "family at fault," is unfavorable to the house staff. This factor is of no practical importance among the obstetricians and "other physicians" for either premature or mature infants.

The frequency of unavoidable disaster among the three groups rendering obstetrical care to the premature infants who died is apparent. However, among the mature infants who died, the frequency of preventability for the obstetrician is lowered by the higher incidence of unavoidable disasters in his experience. It will be recalled that the frequency of preventability associated with unavoidable disaster is negligible.

The fact that there is a higher incidence of unsatisfactory pediatric care associated with the "other physician" group merely reflects the circumstances under which the children were delivered. The patients of the house staff and the obstetrician are more likely to be delivered in an environment

Table XXVI. Frequency of Preventability of Death (Per Cent)—*By Type of Professional Service and by Responsibility Factors*

PREMATURE INFANTS

Responsibility Factors	*Adjusted Totals* House Staff	Obstetricians	Other Physicians
Inadequate prenatal care	53	85*	52*
Errors in medical judgment	78	74	67
Errors in medical technique	77	78	79
Unqualified medical attendant	83*	—	85*
Intercurrent infection	29*	20*	0*
Family at fault	72*	100*	30*
Unavoidable disaster	0	0	1
Unsatisfactory pediatric care	74*	76*	66

* Based on less than 20 deaths.

MATURE INFANTS

Responsibility Factors	*Adjusted Totals* House Staff	Obstetricians	Other Physicians
Inadequate prenatal care	62	71*	69
Errors in medical judgment	84	84	80
Errors in medical technique	85	92*	77
Unqualified medical attendant	100*	100*	83
Intercurrent infection	9*	33*	38*
Family at fault	62*	—	88*
Unavoidable disaster	0	0	3
Unsatisfactory pediatric care	91	69*	81

* Based on less than 20 deaths.

which includes care of the newborn infant by either the pediatric resident staff or a qualified pediatrician, with all the implied advantages of such care. There is a great temptation to assume that this pattern is true for all births, i.e., not only for the perinatal deaths; but there is no information on this point.

These inequalities of distribution help to explain the differences in frequency of preventability for the various sources of obstetrical care.

Table XXVI presents the frequencies of preventability for the premature and mature infants in relation to the type of professional care and the presence of each of the various responsibility factors. No comments are made because of the small number of deaths involved.

TYPE OF HOSPITAL

Table XXVII demonstrates the distribution of the perinatal mortality for both the premature and mature infants according to the type of hospital. It compares types of hospitals and includes deaths in homes.

The usual grouping of hospitals as (1) municipal, (2) voluntary, and (3) proprietary made analysis difficult because there was a lack of homogeneity within groups 1 and 2. In an effort to overcome this obstacle to valid comparison, the following grouping of hospitals has been used:

1. Municipal teaching hospitals
2. Municipal non-teaching hospitals
3. Voluntary teaching hospitals
4. Voluntary non-teaching hospitals
5. Proprietary hospitals

The consistency of the distribution for mature and premature infants is striking. As was shown in Chapter I, the stillbirths of the study appear to be a good cross section of the stillbirths in the city in so far as hospitals are concerned, but the neo-

Table XXVII. Percentage Distribution of Perinatal Deaths—*By Place of Death*

	Adjusted Totals		
Place of Death	Premature	Mature	Total
Municipal teaching hospital	14	13	14
Municipal non-teaching hospital	8	9	9
Voluntary teaching hospital	7	11	9
Voluntary non-teaching hospital	47	47	47
Proprietary hospital	21	19	19
All hospitals	97	99	95
Home deaths	3	1	2
No. of deaths	*477*	*478*	955

Table XXVIII. Frequency of Preventability of Death (Per Cent)—
By Place of Birth

	Adjusted Totals		
Place of Birth	Premature	Mature	Total
Municipal teaching hospital	35	44	39
Municipal non-teaching hospital	36	62	50
Voluntary teaching hospital	18	24	21
Voluntary non-teaching hospital	26	43	35
Proprietary hospital	28	34	31
All hospitals	28	41	35
Home deliveries	56*	79*	62
All deaths†	29	42	35

* Based on less than 20 deaths.
† See Table XIV.

natal deaths in the study do not agree quite so well with the city-wide neonatal deaths.

Table XXVIII is a presentation of the frequency of preventability by place of birth, comparing types of hospitals and including home deliveries. The lowest incidence of preventability is recorded for the voluntary teaching hospitals, the highest for the municipal non-teaching hospitals. The proprietary hospitals are second only to the voluntary teaching hospitals.

In each group, the preventability rates for the teaching hospital are lower than those for the non-teaching institutions. This is true for the deaths of infants of each degree of maturity and for the entire series of deaths in the study as a whole.

For the deaths of premature infants, the differences between teaching and non-teaching hospitals are not significant. However, in the case of mature infants, the difference between the municipal teaching hospitals' figure of 44 per cent and that for the municipal non-teaching hospitals of 62 per cent is statistically significant. Also, for the deaths of mature infants, the difference between the voluntary teaching hospitals (24 per cent) and the voluntary non-teaching hospitals (43 per cent) is significant.

When the populations served by these various types of institutions are considered, the results seem to fall into an understandable pattern. The municipal hospitals are 100 per cent ward care institutions, catering to that segment of the population which carries the highest perinatal mortality rate and which receives the least expert care. Their clientele varies very little between teaching and non-teaching hospitals. Perhaps the better record of the teaching institutions reflects the presence of teaching personnel and of the more highly trained house staffs. Furthermore, the organization of prenatal care, intrapartum procedures, and care of the newborn may be on a higher level in the teaching institutions.

In the voluntary institutions the patients tend to be of the highest economic level, the group in which perinatal mortality rates are lowest. The teaching institutions in this category are affiliated with some of the oldest and best-known medical colleges of the United States. The house staffs are highly selected and the attending staffs caring for private patients comprise mostly qualified specialists.

The populations cared for in the voluntary non-teaching hospitals and the proprietary hospitals tend to be very similar, except for the absence of service patients in the proprietary institutions. It is not surprising, therefore, that there is relatively little difference in the rates for these two groups. It should be borne in mind, however, that these hospitals differ in the following manner: The voluntary non-teaching institutions have better house staffs and auxiliary services, as a rule, but this factor may be overbalanced by the presence of service cases with their greater inherent risks and complications.

This study deals only with fatalities and gives no information concerning infants who survive. An infant must have died to be counted and investigated here. It is possible that an inclusive picture, considering the survivors, might not be consistent with the implications that have been drawn here. Poor practices, inadequate prenatal care, and similar items are recorded only in reference to deaths.

CHAPTER IV

The Relation of Preventability to the Mother

ONE OF THE advantages to be gained from an analysis such as the present one is the opportunity to relate certain characteristics of the mother to the preventability of the deaths. The age, parity, past obstetrical history, and the presence or absence of toxemia are considered here.

AGE AND PARITY

Table XXIX shows the age distribution of the mothers who lost premature or mature infants.

The mothers having premature infants who succumbed

Table XXIX. Percentage Distribution of Perinatal Deaths—*By Age of Mother*

	Adjusted Totals	
Age of Mother	Premature	Mature
Under 15 years	—	0.2*
15–19	5.6	4.2
20–24	23.6	23.5
25–29	25.2	29.8
30–34	15.3	24.7
35–39	17.2	13.2
40–44	5.5	4.0
45–49	1.8*	0.4*
50 or over	1.4*	—
Unknown age	4.4*	—
No. of deaths	*477*	*478*

* Based on less than 20 deaths.

Table XXX. Frequency of Preventability of Death (Per Cent)—
By Age of Mother

	Adjusted Totals	
Age of Mother	Premature	Mature
Under 15 years	—	100*
15–19	43	66
20–24	34	33
25–29	24	43
30–34	35	48
35–39	32	38
40–44	24	36
45–49	0*	33*
50 +	10*	—
Unknown	0*	—
All deaths	29	42

* Based on fewer than 20 deaths.

are somewhat older than those having mature infants who died. Eighty-seven per cent of the mothers who had premature infants who died were under 40, while 96 per cent of those having mature infants who died were under that age. Were it to be assumed that all the women of unknown age (4.4 per cent of the total) were under age 40, there would still be a smaller proportion of women under age 40 bearing the premature infants who succumbed.

For intelligent interpretation, this observation must be related to the distribution of all births by age of the mother.

The frequency of preventability by age of mother for deaths of premature and mature infants is given in Table XXX. The highest frequency of preventability is in the age group 15–19 for deaths of both the premature and the mature infants.

Table XXXI gives the distribution of deaths of premature and mature infants according to age and parity of the mothers. It will be noted that the distribution is essentially the same for both groups of infants.

Table XXXI. Percentage Distribution of Perinatal Deaths—
By Age and Parity of Mother

Age and Parity	*Adjusted Totals* Premature	Mature
UNDER 30 YEARS		
Para 0	33	28
Para 1–4	27	28
Para 5 or more	1	1
Total	61	57
OVER 30 YEARS		
Para 0	7	9
Para 1–4	26	28
Para 5 or more	6	6
Total	39	43
No. of deaths	*477*	*478*

The relationship of preventability to the mothers' age and parity is presented in Table XXXII. Examination of Table XXXII reveals that there is a higher percentage of preventability for para 0, regardless of the infant's maturity and regardless of the age of the mother. This difference is slight for

Table XXXII. Frequency of Preventability of Death (Per Cent)—
By Age and Parity of Mother

Age and Parity	*Adjusted Totals* Premature	Mature
UNDER 30 YEARS		
Para 0	28	50
Para 1–4	26	33
Para 5 or more	1*	12*
All deaths under 30	27	40
OVER 30 YEARS		
Para 0	40	52
Para 1–4	26	38
Para 5 or more	44*	57*
All deaths over 30	31	43
All deaths†	29	42

* Based on less than 22 deaths.
† See Table XIV.

the premature infants whose mothers were under 30, but is marked for the older group, both as to maturity status and as to parity of mother. The numbers of deaths among babies of mothers of para 5 or more, over age 30, are only 20 and 21, respectively, for the premature and mature infants, and were therefore not considered in the comparison.

In all subdivisions of Table XXXII the frequency of preventability is greater for the mature infants than for the premature ones. This general finding, greater preventability for mature than for premature infants, was discussed in Chapter II.

MATERNAL COMPLICATIONS

The frequency of many of the maternal complications, such as contracted pelvis, tuberculosis, diabetes, heart disease, acute infectious diseases, and similar conditions, is so small that tabulation and consideration of them gives no worthwhile information. Threatened abortion during the existing pregnancy, however, was recorded rather frequently. Table XXXIII demonstrates that 11.1 per cent of the deaths among premature infants were associated with threatened abortion as compared with only 6.1 per cent of the deaths among the mature infants. There is apparent a pattern of greater frequency of threatened abortion in mothers whose infants were born prematurely than in those who bore full-

Table XXXIII. Frequency of Threatened Abortion—
For 955 Perinatal Deaths

Degree of Maturity	*A*		*B*		*C*		*Adjusted Total, %*
	No.	%	No.	%	No.	%	
Premature	6	5.4	47	16.8	13	14.7	11.1
Mature	9	7.0	10	4.9	7	4.7	6.1
All degrees	15	6.3	57	11.8	20	8.5	8.6

term babies. In order to assess properly the role of threatened abortion in premature termination of pregnancy and in order to evaluate the importance of this finding in the increase of the neonatal mortality rate it would be necessary to have this information also for infants who did not die in the neonatal period.

PAST OBSTETRICAL EXPERIENCE

Table XXXIV records the past obstetrical experience of the mothers. They are grouped according to the category of their loss (i.e., A, B, and C groups of premature and mature infants) in the present study, although all the data in the table refer to their previous pregnancies. The table reveals that there is no significant difference between the past obstetrical experience of mothers who had premature or mature infants in the present study (see first and second sections of the table). Therefore a combination of the data on premature and mature deaths (see third section of the table) was used as the basis of the discussion that follows.

The frequency of abortions in previous pregnancies is the same for the A and C categories, but is significantly higher for the B category. The frequencies for categories A and C are quite close to the generally accepted value of 10 per cent, but the B frequency, 21 per cent, is significantly different from the accepted figure.

Examination of the frequencies of previous stillbirths and previous neonatal deaths seems to indicate the possibility of a perinatal loss pattern for the patients. The A patients have lost 15 per cent of their previous viable pregnancies, the B patients 10 per cent and the C patients 7 per cent. These differences are statistically significant. The ratio of stillbirths to neonatal deaths in previous pregnancies also varies from cate-

Table XXXIV. Past Obstetrical History of Mothers—
By Category of Infant in Present Study

MOTHERS OF PREMATURE INFANTS

Data on Previous Pregnancy	*Category of Death in Present Study* A	B	C
No. of women	110	279	88
Women with previous pregnancies	62	165	47
Previous pregnancies	148	423	101
Viable pregnancies	131 (89%)	329 (78%)	88 (87%)
Abortions	17 (11%)	94 (22%)	13 (13%)
Perinatal deaths	18 (14%)	35 (11%)	4 (5%)
Stillbirths	5	12	2
Neonatal deaths	13	23	2
Average no. of pregnancies per patient	2.4	2.6	2.1
Average no. of viable pregnancies per patient	2.1	2.0	1.9

MOTHERS OF MATURE INFANTS

	A	B	C
No. of women	127	204	147
Women with previous pregnancies	77	131	94
Previous pregnancies	231	315	217
Viable pregnancies	202 (87%)	257 (72%)	189 (87%)
Abortions	29 (13%)	58 (18%)	28 (13%)
Perinatal deaths	29 (14%)	23 (9%)	14 (7%)
Stillbirths	20	11	4
Neonatal deaths	9	12	10
Average no. of pregnancies per patient	3.0	2.4	2.3
Average no. of viable pregnancies per patient	2.6	2.0	2.0

MOTHERS OF PREMATURE AND MATURE INFANTS, COMBINED

	A	B	C
No. of women	237	483	235
Women with previous pregnancies	139	296	141
Previous pregnancies	379	738	318
Viable pregnancies	333 (88%)	586 (79%)	277 (87%)
Abortions	46 (12%)	152 (21%)	41 (13%)
Perinatal deaths	47 (15%)	58 (10%)	18 (7%)
Stillbirths	25	23	6
Neonatal deaths	22	35	12
Average no. of pregnancies per patient	2.7	2.3	2.1
Average no. of viable pregnancies per patient	2.4	2.0	2.0

gory to category. Among the A's, approximately 50 per cent of the previous perinatal deaths were stillbirths; among the B's well under one-half were stillbirths; and among the C's, only about 33 per cent were stillbirths. However, no statistical significance may be attached to this distribution of stillbirths in previous pregnancies.

TOXEMIAS OF PREGNANCY

Table XXXV shows the frequency of toxemias of pregnancy in each category for premature and mature infants. The table reveals that 17 per cent of the deaths of premature infants and 15 per cent of the deaths of mature infants were associated with toxemia of pregnancy. Such a high incidence of toxemia is far above that which would be observed in a large series of births in New York City. In one large municipal hospital only 9 per cent of all births were associated with toxemias of pregnancy; this difference is more striking in the light of the fact that 75 per cent of this hospital's clientele is made up of Negroes, in whom toxemias would be expected to be more prevalent than among the white women.[1] There appears to be a concentration of toxemias in the A category for the deaths of both the premature and the mature infants.

Table XXXV. Frequency of Toxemia of Pregnancy (Per Cent)—
For 955 Perinatal Deaths

Degree of Maturity	*A*	*B*	*C*	*Adjusted Total*
Premature	22	13	15	17
Mature	18	12	6	15
All toxemia deaths	20	12	9	16

[1] *Annual Reports.* State University of New York College of Medicine, Department of Obstetrics and Gynecology. 1951–1953.

Table XXXVI. Frequency of Preventability of Death (Per Cent)—
Toxemia of Pregnancy

PREMATURE INFANTS

	A	*B*	*C*	*Adjusted Total*
Toxemia	54	39	31*	48
No toxemia	14	31	56	25
All deaths†	23	32	52	29

* Based on fewer than 20 deaths.
† See Table XIV.

MATURE INFANTS

	A	*B*	*C*	*Adjusted Total*
Toxemia	61	54	56*	59
No toxemia	29	52	44	39
All deaths†	35	53	45	42

* Based on fewer than 20 deaths.
† See Table XIV.

Table XXXVI presents the frequency of deaths that were preventable in premature and mature infants, respectively, which were or were not associated with toxemia of pregnancy. Among the deaths of premature infants it will be noted that there is a considerable concentration of preventability in the A category. The preventability in this category for stillbirths associated with toxemia is four times that for the premature stillbirths not associated with toxemia of pregnancy. Upon moving into the B category prematures, one notes that the frequencies of preventability in cases of toxemia and cases without toxemia approach equality. While the frequency of preventability among the C prematures is based on few cases, it is still apparent that there is a reversal of the pattern of preventability seen in the A category, as regards presence or absence of toxemia.

The deaths of mature infants show a pattern similar to that just described. Among the stillbirths the difference previ-

Table XXXVII. Frequency of Toxemia (Per Cent)—
By Type of Professional Service

	Adjusted Totals	
Type of Service	Premature	Mature
House staff	23.6	19.1
Obstetricians	12.9	10.2
Other physicians	18.2	15.3
Unknown care	10.0	9.2
All services	17.4	14.8

ously mentioned is not so marked, but it is present. It seems apparent that the B and C categories, with regard to preventability, are not particularly influenced by the presence of toxemias of pregnancy. The fact that preventability looms so large among the cases with toxemias in the stillbirth category suggests, in the opinion of the panels, that antenatal care was often less than expert.

Table XXXVII demonstrates the frequency of toxemia of pregnancy for each type of professional service for the premature and mature infants, respectively. The highest frequency of toxemia is found among those patients who received care by house staffs. The next highest frequency of toxemia is for other physicians, and the lowest is for the obstetricians. This pattern is consistent for both the premature and the mature infants. Prenatal care and the economic status of the populations cared for by each group undoubtedly are closely related to the frequencies recorded in Table XXXVII. Knowledge of the frequency of toxemias among all births, by type of professional care, would be a useful datum. This would allow the calculation of perinatal mortality rates specific for each type of professional service; then better evaluation of the obstetrical care could be obtained than is possible from the present study. Table XXXVII also illustrates how the house staff experience is loaded with a complication having a high frequency of preventability. This is one of the factors previously alluded to as contributing to the high preventability frequency among infants cared for by a house staff.

CHAPTER V

Analgesia and Anesthesia

In March 1847 there appeared in the British *Monthly Journal of Medical Science* an article entitled, "Notes on the Employment of the Inhalation of Sulfuric Ether in the Practice of Midwifery," by Dr. James Y. Simpson. In 1902 Steinbuckel introduced "twilight sleep," and in 1906 Gauss reported on 1000 cases treated with "twilight sleep" in labor.

Since those early workers reported their results, the obstetricians have found it either necessary or expedient to use analgesic and anesthetic agents in the conduct of labor. There is no doubt that the use of these agents has made the process of childbirth a quieter and more acceptable experience. Continuous attempts have been made to evaluate their influence upon the course of labor, delivery, and the fetus.

This chapter is concerned with an attempt to determine whether the use of analgesia and anesthesia is associated with stillbirths and neonatal deaths.

Table XXXVIII indicates the frequency of the use of various types of analgesia.

More than half of the deliveries of the premature infants were conducted under some analgesic agent (50.8 per cent). The frequency of use of analgesia is approximately the same for all categories. For the mature infants, the frequency of the administration of analgesic agents during labor was

Table XXXVIII. Percentage Distribution of Perinatal Deaths—
By Analgesic Agent

	Adjusted Totals	
Agent	Premature	Mature
Unknown	8	5
None	41	35
Barbiturate	3*	2*
Barbiturate and Demerol	3*	4
Barbiturate and Scopolamine	1*	0*
Barbiturate, Scopolamine, and Demerol	2*	3*
Scopolamine	3*	2*
Scopolamine and Demerol	17	28
Demerol	21	19
Others	1*	2*
No. of deaths	*477*	*478*

* Based on less than 20 deaths.

found to be at least 60.2 per cent. Here, too, the frequency is approximately the same for all categories.

Table XXXIX records the frequency of preventability for premature and mature infants, respectively, according to the analgesic agent used. Because of the small numbers involved, no conclusions are drawn from these tables.

It was not possible to record and analyze the data for the interval between the last administration of analgesia and birth. While the analgesic agent used was unknown in less than 10 per cent of the deaths of premature infants and 7 per cent of the mature infants, the interval between administration and delivery is unknown in many of the cases.

In Table XL are recorded the percentages of deaths of premature and mature infants that were associated with various types of anesthetic. The pattern is surprisingly similar in both groups. The basic data show that inhalation anesthesia was most frequent in categories B and C. Without information on the use of these agents in all births, it cannot be concluded that the low frequency of local and conduction

Table XXXIX. Frequency of Preventability of Death (Per Cent)—
By Analgesic Agent

PREMATURE INFANTS

Agent	*A*	*B*	*C*	*Adjusted Total*
Unknown agent	13*	29*	50*	17
None	18	29	50	25.6
Barbiturate	50*	10*	—	22*
Barbiturate and Demerol	33*	72*	100*	53*
Barbiturate and Scopolamine	—	33*	—	33*
Barbiturate and Scopolamine and Demerol	50*	40*	0.0*	42*
Scopolamine	50*	46*	100.0*	44*
Scopolamine and Demerol	14	42	44	28
Demerol	36	30	61*	35
Others	—	0.0*	—	0
All deaths†	23	32	52	29

* Based on less than 20 deaths.
† See Table XIV.

MATURE INFANTS

Agent	*A*	*B*	*C*	*Adjusted Total*
Unknown agent	63*	25*	70*	59
None	20	49	52	32
Barbiturate	0.0*	25*	72*	24*
Barbiturate and Demerol	50*	60*	0.0*	53*
Barbiturate and Scopolamine	—	0*	0*	0*
Barbiturate and Scopolamine and Demerol	100*	58*	—	77
Scopolamine	0*	0*	67*	7*
Scopolamine and Demerol	47	56	39	49
Demerol	30	61	33	42
Others	50*	33*	25*	39
All deaths†	35	53	45	42

* Based on less than 20 deaths.
† See Table XIV.

anesthesia indicates that these methods are superior for the premature infant. It is probably true that more premature deliveries are conducted under inhalation anesthesia than under any other type, in spite of contrary opinions of many obstetricians and pediatricians interested in the subject.

The fact that inhalation anesthesia was most frequently employed for the mothers of mature infants who died was

Table XL. Percentage Distribution of Perinatal Deaths—
By Type of Anesthetic Agent Used for Delivery

	Adjusted Total	
Type of Agent	Premature	Mature
None	29	18
Inhalation	47	54
Intravenous	1*	0*
Local	6	11
Conduction	7	10
Unknown	9	7
No. of deaths	*477*	*478*

* Based on fewer than 20 deaths.

to be anticipated; it is probably the type most frequently used for all deliveries. It is of interest to note that 21 per cent of the mature infants who died had been delivered under local or conduction anesthesia.

The frequency of preventability, as shown in Table XLI, appears not to have been influenced by the anesthetic agent administered. The difference in the frequency of preventability between no anesthesia and inhalation anesthesia is very small for the premature deaths. The observed difference for the mature infants (7 per cent) is not significant.

The largest disparity between frequency of preventability for no anesthesia and inhalation anesthesia is in the C category for both mature and premature infants. This is probably related to the fact that the causes of death in category C are unlikely to be directly associated with either analgesic agents, anesthetic agents, or the actual conduct of the delivery. Rather, the causes of death are likely to be associated with disease or lack of pediatric care.

It is certain that analgesia and anesthesia are of importance in the successful conduct of a delivery for both mother and child. This association is always difficult to evaluate. In a study restricted to deaths and not specifically designed for

Table XLI. Frequency of Preventability of Death (Per Cent)—
By Anesthetic Agent

PREMATURE INFANTS

Type of Agent	*A*	*B*	*C*	*Adjusted Total*
None	24	23	80	26
Inhalation	21	39	46	29
Intravenous	—	50*	—	50*
Local	—	24	39*	26
Conduction	40*	39	50*	40
Unknown	18*	33	44*	27
All deaths†	23	32	52	29

* Based on less than 20 deaths.
† See Table XIV.

MATURE INFANTS

Type of Agent	*A*	*B*	*C*	*Adjusted Total*
None	25	62	55	42
Inhalation	27	52	38	35
Intravenous	—	0*	—	0*
Local	77*	64	44*	69
Conduction	55*	30	38*	42
Unknown	33*	58*	64*	45
All deaths†	35	53	45	42

* Based on less than 20 deaths.
† See Table XIV.

the purpose of evaluating analgesia and anesthesia, it is almost impossible to draw conclusions concerning the effect of these agents upon perinatal mortality.

CHAPTER VI

Method of Delivery

THE METHOD of delivery and the presentation of the infant at delivery are currently thought to be of decreasing importance in perinatal mortality. It has been stated recently that birth trauma as a cause of perinatal mortality is on the decline. This could not be substantiated in the present investigation, in which birth trauma was found to be an appreciable and important cause of death. This is discussed in Chapter VIII, "Causes of Death." It was deemed of significance to investigate the relationship of the presentation and the method of delivery to perinatal mortality.

PRESENTATION

Table XLII shows the distribution of the perinatal mortality by presentation at delivery, for the premature and the mature infants, respectively. In a series including all births one would anticipate a frequency of from 7 to 9 per cent of "abnormal" presentations. In this series of perinatal deaths, the frequency of such presentations is 28 per cent for the premature infants and 14 per cent for the mature infants.

High death rates are associated with presentations other than vertex. The breech presented in approximately 23 per cent of the deaths of premature infants in this study, as compared with an incidence of 4 per cent of breech presenta-

Table XLII. Percentage Distribution of Perinatal Deaths—
By Presentation

Presentation	*Adjusted Totals* Premature	Mature
Vertex anterior	58	63
Vertex posterior	8	14
Vertex rotated	2	8
Breech, frank	17	8
Breech, full	1	1
Breech, footling	5	2
Face or brow	2	2
Transverse lie	3	1
Compound	0	0
Unknown	4	1
No. of deaths	*477*	*478*

tions in a series of 845 premature deliveries in a large New York City hospital.[1]

Among the perinatal deaths of mature infants there was a frequency of breech presentations of approximately 11 per cent; in a similar series of 5250 consecutive deliveries at a large New York City hospital, the incidence of breech presentations was only 2 per cent.[2] As recorded in Table XLII, the frequency of "transverse lie" is also higher among the infants than the expected incidence of 0.5 per cent to 1 per cent reported by many institutions for all births.

These observations emphasize the high mortality rates associated with the abnormal presentations.

It would appear from Table XLIII that the presence of an occiput posterior and consequent corrective manipulations of vertex (rotation) carries a higher frequency of preventability than a normal occiput anterior. This is true for the deaths of both the premature and mature infants. Because

[1] *Annual Reports*. Department of Obstetrics and Gynecology, State University of New York, 1951–1953.

[2] *Ibid.*

of the small numbers involved, conclusions concerning the abnormal positions cannot be drawn with assurance.

Table XLIII. Frequency of Preventability of Death (Per Cent)—*By Presentation*

PREMATURE INFANTS

Presentation	*A*	*B*	*C*	*Adjusted Total*
Vertex anterior	22	30	54	27
Vertex posterior	0*	39	—	33
Vertex rotated	50*	72*	100*	64*
Breech, frank	25	23	18*	24
Breech, full	—	0*	100*	8*
Breech, footling	25*	41*	75*	37
Face or brow	0*	0*	100*	4*
Transverse lie	50*	63*	0*	54*
Compound	—	0*	0*	0*
Unknown	20*	50*	100*	31*
All deaths†	23	32	52	29

* Based on less than 20 deaths.
† See Table XIV.

MATURE INFANTS

Presentation	*A*	*B*	*C*	*Adjusted Total*
Vertex anterior	27	38	46	32
Vertex posterior	72*	68	50*	69
Vertex rotated	73*	57*	50*	67
Breech, frank	17*	60*	0*	29
Breech, full	100*	50*	—	73*
Breech, footling	100*	72*	—	67*
Face or brow	50*	50*	—	50*
Transverse lie	50*	100*	50*	53*
Compound	—	—	0*	0*
Unknown	—	67*	50*	67*
All deaths†	35	53	45	42

* Based on less than 20 deaths.
† See Table XIV.

METHOD OF DELIVERY

Table XLIV shows the frequency of the various types of operative delivery in the deaths of premature and mature infants. The fact that the frequency of operative deliveries

Table XLIV. Percentage Distribution of Perinatal Deaths—
By Method of Delivery

Method of Delivery	*Adjusted Totals* Premature	Mature
Spontaneous vertex	47	45
Spontaneous breech	7	3
Low forceps	12	21
Mid forceps	1	10
High forceps	0	1
Cesarean section	15	11
Cesarean section after high forceps	0	0
Version and extraction	2	2
Version followed by destructive operation	0	0
Breech extraction	14	6
Breech extraction and destructive operation	1	1
Unknown	1	0
No. of deaths	*477*	*478*

is 46 per cent for the deaths of premature infants and 52 per cent for the deaths of the mature infants, as contrasted with a more or less standard figure of approximately 30 per cent for all births, is again an indication of the higher mortality associated with operative deliveries.

The foregoing observation well illustrates the fact that the frequency of any circumstance among deaths may differ from the frequency among all births. Another illustrative comparison is the frequency of cesarean section: 15 per cent among the premature group and 11 per cent among the mature group, as compared with an estimated frequency of 4 per cent in all deliveries.[3]

In our sample of almost 1000 perinatal deaths (237 stillbirths), four destructive operations were performed. These were equally divided between the premature infants and the mature infants. Since our sample contains approximately 10 per cent of all stillbirths that occurred in New York City

[3] N. J. Eastman, *Obstetrics.* 10th Edition. Appleton-Century-Crofts, New York, 1950. P. 1101.

in the period under study, one might assume that some 40 infants were so delivered in New York City in 1950. Examination of the records of the four cases mentioned reveals that two of these operations were performed upon infants who had died in utero prior to the onset of labor. This means of delivery was used to ease the process for the mother.

On four occasions unsuccessful attempts were made to deliver with high forceps, and then the physician resorted to cesarean section. Unfortunately, there is no information about the frequency of this procedure for all New York City births. Obstetricians consider the application of high forceps unwise. When it is attempted unsuccessfully and cesarean section is performed, it may be concluded that obstetrical judgment was inferior. The Committee was of this opinion and declared these deaths preventable.

The basic data show that cesarean section was most frequent in category B; 20 per cent of the premature and 15 per cent of the mature babies who died were so delivered. Breech extractions were concentrated in categories A and B for both the premature and mature infants. Thus it appears that certain types of delivery may be closely associated with stillbirths and early neonatal deaths. Perhaps this is a causal relationship. The cause of death in the A and B categories is likely to be associated with the conduct of labor or method of delivery, while the deaths in the C category are likely to be associated with non-controllable prenatal and pediatric factors.

Table XLV presents the frequency of preventability according to the method of delivery for the various categories. More than 40 per cent of the deaths of infants delivered by cesarean section were held to have been preventable. This does not reflect credit on the use of this operation. Sometimes

Table XLV. Frequency of Preventability of Death (Per Cent)—
By Method of Delivery

PREMATURE INFANTS

Method of Delivery	*A*	*B*	*C*	*Adjusted Total*
Spontaneous vertex	17	27	61	25
Spontaneous breech	13*	17*	63*	18*
Low forceps	17*	28	39*	24
Mid forceps	100*	75*	100*	88*
High forceps	—	—	—	—
Cesarean section	31*	48	33*	42
Cesarean section after high forceps	100*	—	—	100*
Version and extraction	33*	40*	100*	36*
Version followed by destructive operation	100*	—	—	100*
Breech extraction	33*	30	0*	31
Breech extraction and destructive operation	0*	—	—	0*
Unknown	0*	—	0*	0*
All deaths†	23	32	52	29

* Based on less than 20 deaths.
† See Table XIV.

MATURE INFANTS

Method of Delivery	*A*	*B*	*C*	*Adjusted Total*
Spontaneous vertex	24	50	53	36
Spontaneous breech	0*	100*	0*	80*
Low forceps	25	45	32	34
Mid forceps	74*	65*	33*	67
High forceps	100*	100*	—	100*
Cesarean section	42*	45	64*	44
Cesarean section after high forceps	100*	—	—	100*
Version and extraction	50*	100*	—	54*
Version followed by destructive operation	—	—	—	—
Breech extraction	27*	0*	—	23*
Breech extraction and destructive operation	50*	—	—	50
Unknown	100*	—	—	100*
All deaths†	35	53	45	42

* Based on less than 20 deaths.
† See Table XIV.

it was employed too late, sometimes too early, and sometimes when not indicated. The anesthetic agent for the operation often was not chosen with wisdom nor with consideration for the age and condition of mother and infant.

This study would seem to confirm the previously published condemnation of the difficult mid-forceps operation. It will be noted that this operation was attended by a high frequency of preventability for all categories.

The preventability rate for breech extractions is so similar to that for spontaneous deliveries that one cannot criticize the performance of this maneuver.

A sample of all births classified by maturity, type of delivery, and presentation is clearly needed for a better interpretation than can be given here of the effects of these factors on perinatal mortality.

CHAPTER VII

Time of Death

THE TIME of death was recorded for all deaths in the study. Whether death occurred before or during labor is recorded in Table XLVI for the stillborn infants, and the time of death in the neonatal period is shown in Tables XLIX and LI.

STILLBIRTHS

Table XLVI reveals that death during labor occurs twice as frequently in the mature stillborn infants as in those born prematurely. This difference is significant.

In Table XLVII the relationship between the time of death and the time of delivery is shown. In this study no appreciable difference was noted between the premature and the mature infants with respect to the interval between death and delivery.

Thirty-five per cent of the 17 premature deaths at less than one hour prior to delivery were considered preventable, whereas in the 25 deaths of mature infants occurring at the same time, the preventability rate rose to 68 per cent. This difference is of borderline significance.

The general preventability rate for stillborn premature infants dying intrapartum is slightly higher than the rate for those dying before labor. For the mature infants, however, the rate is much higher for those dying during labor than for

Table XLVI. Time of Death—*Stillbirths*

Time of Death	*Premature* No.	*Premature* %	*Mature* No.	*Mature* %
Before labor	84	76	69	54
During labor	26	24	58	46
No. of deaths	*110*	*100*	*127*	*100*

Table XLVII. Time Between Death and Delivery—*Stillbirths*

Length of Time	*Premature* No.	*Premature* %	*Mature* No.	*Mature* %
Less than 30 minutes	12	11	19	15
30–60 minutes	5	4	6	5
60–120 minutes	0	0	5	4
120–180 minutes	1	1	8	6
180–240 minutes	1	1	1	1
Over 240 minutes	68	62	67	53
Unknown	23	21	21	16
No. of deaths	*110*	*100*	*127*	*100*

Table XLVIII. Frequency of Preventability of Death (Per Cent)—*By Time of Death: Stillbirths*

Time of Death	*Premature*	*Mature*
Before labor	19	12
During labor	35	62
All deaths*	23	35

* See Table XIV.

those dying antepartum. Apparently the time of death influences the determination of preventability to a greater degree in the mature infants than in the premature.

The basic data from which Table XLVIII was prepared reveal that in 75 per cent of the non-preventable stillbirths, regardless of maturity, death occurred before labor. On the other hand, 64 per cent of the preventable premature stillbirths occurred during labor, but only 18 per cent of the preventable deaths of mature infants occurred prior to labor.

Table XLIX. Time of Death—*Early Neonatal Deaths*

Time of Death	*Premature* No.	*Premature* %	*Mature* No.	*Mature* %
First 12 hours	127	46	69	34
12–24 hours	45	16	30	15
24–48 hours	69	25	51	25
48–72 hours	21	7	32	15
1–5 days	17	6	22	11
No. of deaths	*279*	*100*	*204*	*100*

Table L. Frequency of Preventability of Death (Per Cent)—
By Time of Death: Early Neonatal Deaths

Time of Death	*Premature*	*Mature*
First 12 hours	35	47
12–24 hours	36	64
24–48 hours	31	61
48–72 hours	10*	47
1–5 days	35	46
All deaths†	32	53

* Based on only 21 deaths.
† See Table XIV.

EARLY NEONATAL DEATHS

Table XLIX gives the distribution of early neonatal deaths for both the premature and mature infants according to the time of death.

Table L gives the preventability rate in relation to time of early neonatal death for both premature and mature infants. For the early neonatal deaths among premature infants, there is an amazing similarity in the percentages of preventability for all times of death. A similar consistency is demonstrated for the mature infants.

The data indicate that the time of death was of no significance in the determination of preventability of early neonatal deaths.

Table LI. Time of Death—*Late Neonatal Deaths*

	Premature		*Mature*	
Time of Death	No.	%	No.	%
6–10 days	50	57	60	41
10–30 days	38	43	87	59
No. of deaths	*88*	*100*	*147*	*100*

Table LII. Frequency of Preventability of Death (Per Cent)—
By Time of Death: Late Neonatal Deaths

Time of Death	*Premature*	*Mature*
6–10 days	42	50
10–30 days	66	41
All deaths*	52	45

* See Table XIV.

LATE NEONATAL DEATHS

In Table LI is given the distribution of late neonatal deaths by time of death for both premature and mature infants.

Table LII gives the frequency of preventability by time of late neonatal death for both premature and mature infants. The high frequency of preventability for the premature infants dying in the period from 10 to 30 days was to be expected in view of the frequency of unsatisfactory pediatric care for the premature infants, as shown in Chapter II.

These data for deaths do not necessarily reflect rates and chances of dying. Tabulation of all births would be necessary to provide this information.

CHAPTER VIII

Causes of Death

THE DETERMINATION and evaluation of the causes of death are among the prime purposes of this study and analysis.

In the study there were available two or three sources of information on the causes of death. For the infants submitted to postmortem examination there were three categories of causes:

1. Pathologic causes as determined by the author and the Editorial Committee after a study of the records, including autopsies.
2. Clinical causes as recorded on the hospital charts.
3. Causes recorded on death or stillbirth certificates.

For the cases in which autopsies were not performed, only the last two categories of causes were available.

PATHOLOGIC CAUSES

It will be recalled that autopsies were performed in only 413 of the deaths studied. The frequency of autopsies in the several categories is shown in Table LIII.

Table LIII. Frequency of Autopsies (Per Cent)—
For 955 Perinatal Deaths

	A	*B*	*C*	*Adjusted Total*
Premature	17	44	52	31
Mature	29	53	54	40
All deaths	24	47	54	35

The pathologic causes of death were determined by the author and the Editorial Committee on the basis of the pathologic data available; that is, the results of the post-mortem examination as originally recorded by the hospital pathologist on the hospital chart, together with any supplementary data assembled during the re-examination of the records. In many instances the new information made possible a more accurate statement of the cause of death.

Prematurity was excluded from the causes found at autopsy and those recorded on the hospital charts. Whenever prematurity was listed as a cause of death, the author and the Editorial Committee restudied the case and selected the best diagnosis that they could make from the records. This exclusion was necessary because prematurity tends to become a "wastebasket" in which demonstrable causes may be lost.

For those cases submitted to autopsy, the pathologic causes are tabulated in Table LIV.

Because of the small number of cases in which autopsies were performed in the A category (19 premature and 37 mature infants) and because of the large number of "unknown causes," no confident statements may be made about the frequency of the various causes of death in category A.

It was gratifying to be able to demonstrate that "unknown cause" occurred with negligible frequency in categories B and C. Only in category A, premature and mature, was a higher frequency recorded: 53 per cent and 41 per cent, respectively. Even in category A the cause of death could be assigned in 50 per cent or more of the cases in which there were autopsies. This outcome is particularly pleasing when it is realized that these autopsies were performed in many different hospitals with varying orientations toward perinatal mortality and varying interest in the prob-

Table LIV. Percentage Distribution of Deaths—
By Pathologic Causes

PREMATURE INFANTS

Causes	*A*	*B*	*C*
Birth trauma	11	13	13
Anoxia	26	6	—
Malformations	—	11	20
Infections	5	6	39
Hemolytic diseases	—	5	6
Pulmonary pathology	5	54	13
Unknown and others	53	5	9
Not autopsied	83	56	48

MATURE INFANTS

Causes	*A*	*B*	*C*
Birth trauma	11	21	2
Anoxia	30	4	—
Malformations	—	27	26
Infections	5	4	53
Hemolytic diseases	13	16	9
Pulmonary pathology	—	26	9
Unknown and others	41	2	1
Not autopsied	72	47	46

lem. The results would seem to refute assertions to the effect that autopsies on stillborn and newborn infants are futile.

The following conclusions seem justified from Table LIV:

1. Birth trauma causes death with equal frequency in all the categories of premature births. It would be logical to suppose that birth trauma would occur less frequently in category C than in A or B. It is possible, of course, that bias in the selection of the babies for autopsy is responsible for the equality actually found, and that had there been autopsies in more cases, this equality would not obtain. In the mature infants the anticipated pattern was more nearly approached, as 11 per cent of the A, 21 per cent of the B, and only 2 per cent of the C deaths were classified as due to birth trauma.

The frequency with which birth trauma was responsible for stillbirths was equal in the mature and the premature infants. The following specific items are included under "birth trauma":

Intracranial hemorrhage with tear of the tentorium
Intracranial hemorrhage with tear of the falx
Intracranial hemorrhage with tear of the falx and tentorium
Intracranial hemorrhage without tear of dura
Intraventricular hemorrhage
Subarachnoid hemorrhage
Rupture of the liver
Rupture of other organ or viscus
Spinal cord injury
Injury of larynx
Adrenal injury

2. Anoxia was judged responsible for about the same percentage of stillbirths among the premature as among the mature infants (26 per cent and 30 per cent, respectively). Likewise, among early neonatal deaths and late neonatal deaths, anoxia was responsible with equal frequency in both premature and mature infants. It might have been anticipated that this cause would account for a greater percentage of the deaths.

The following were included under "anoxia":

Abruptio placentae
Marginal sinus rupture
Placenta previa
Prolapse of the cord
Rupture of a cord vessel
"Other" cord obstruction
Toxemia
Uterine inertia
Diabetes
Abnormal uterine contraction
Rupture of the uterus
Intrapartum infection
Prolonged second stage of labor (no trauma)
Death of the mother
Maternal medication
Cardiac failure in the mother

3. Malformations caused no stillbirths among either premature or mature infants. Malformations, however, did contribute appreciably to the causes of death in the B and C categories, regardless of state of maturity. A greater proportion of the deaths of mature infants was caused by malformations than was true for the premature infants. It might have been expected that malformations would account for a greater proportion of early neonatal deaths than of late neonatal deaths, but such was not the case.

Only major malformations which were deemed to be incompatible with life were included.

4. Infections were responsible for a greater proportion of deaths in group C than in group B. There was a higher frequency in the C mature infants than in the C premature group.

The specific entities included in this group were:

Pneumonia	Meningitis
Omphalitis	Peritonitis
Septicemia	Diarrhea

Syphilis

5. Hemolytic diseases were not responsible for any premature stillbirths. The occurrence of hemolytic disease was more frequent in the mature than in the premature infants. That many of these babies are edematous causes them to be relatively heavy for their gestational age, a fact which tends to shift them into the category of mature infants. This is especially likely for those who die. Of the 33 deaths from hemolytic diseases in categories B and C (premature and mature), 13 were called preventable.

The deaths from hemolytic diseases were caused almost exclusively by erythroblastosis fetalis. There is a scattering of cases of hemorrhagic disease of the newborn.

6. Pulmonary pathology was the responsible factor in over 50 per cent of the B premature deaths. This category consists largely of deaths from atelectasis with or without hyaline material. Microscopic examination revealed hyaline membranes in one-third of the cases in this category.

This group of conditions consists of:

Atelectasis with hyaline membranes
Atelectasis without hyaline membranes
Aspiration

In Table LV the causes of death determined at autopsy are correlated with the type of professional service. This is done for the premature and the mature infants separately. Analysis of Table LV produces no definite result because of the small number of autopsies. The table is presented merely to illustrate a potentially profitable type of analysis, were sufficient data available.

CLINICAL CAUSES

The foregoing discussion has been limited to a consideration of only 35.4 per cent of all the cases, because that was the proportion in which autopsies were performed. In order to evaluate causes of death for the entire sample of 955 deaths, either the causes of death written on the hospital chart, the clinical causes, or those on the death certificate must be tabulated (Table LVI and Table LVII). As will be subsequently shown, the clinical causes appear to be more reliable than do the causes on the death certificate.

The clinical causes are presented in Table LVI. Within sampling error, this picture reflects the causes of death, category by category, for New York City's perinatal mortality in the period under study.

Table LV. Percentage Distribution of Perinatal Deaths—*By Pathologic Causes of Death and by Type of Professional Service*

PREMATURE INFANTS

	A			*B*			*C*		
	House Staff	Obste-trician	Other Phys.	House Staff	Obste-trician	Other Phys.	House Staff	Obste-trician	Other Phys
Birth trauma	20	0	14	10	19	8	20	15	10
Anoxia	20	0	57	8	6	3	0	0	0
Congenital malformations	0	0	0	10	9	15	26	15	20
Infections	20	0	0	8	3	8	40	31	50
Hemolytic diseases	0	0	0	3	3	15	7	8	10
Pulmonary pathology	0	16	0	61	50	43	7	15	0
Unknown and others	40	84	29	0	10	8	0	15	0
Autopsied deaths									
No.	5	6	7	39	32	26	15	13	10
Per cent	19	40	13	54	49	28	63	50	46

Table LV (*continued*)

MATURE INFANTS

	A			B			C		
	House Staff	Obste-trician	Other Phys.	House Staff	Obste-trician	Other Phys.	House Staff	Obste-trician	Other Phys.
Birth trauma	19	0	9	24	11	19	0	0	4
Anoxia	37	50	0	14	0	0	0	0	0
Congenital malformations	0	0	0	14	46	26	31	29	27
Infections	0	10	0	0	0	7	52	53	41
Hemolytic diseases	19	0	27	10	25	17	10	12	9
Pulmonary pathology	0	0	0	31	18	31	7	0	18
Unknown and others	25	40	64	7	0	0	0	6	0
Autopsied deaths									
No.	16	10	11	29	28	42	29	17	22
Per cent	34	33	27	62	67	46	63	57	42

Table LVI. Percentage Distribution of Perinatal Deaths—
By Clinical Causes

PREMATURE INFANTS

Cause of Death	A	B	C
Birth trauma	4	9	10
Anoxia	49	11	0
Malformations	5	9	13
Infections	4	4	31
Hemolytic diseases	2	3	9
Pulmonary pathology	1	60	34
Unknown and others	35	4	3
Total	100	100	100

MATURE INFANTS

Cause of Death	A	B	C
Birth trauma	11	25	5
Anoxia	46	7	1
Malformations	7	25	31
Infections	0	5	39
Hemolytic diseases	4	12	10
Pulmonary pathology	0	19	7
Unknown and others	32	7	7
Total	100	100	100

DEATH CERTIFICATES

Table LVII presents the causes recorded on death certificates for the premature and mature infants, respectively.

Comparison between causes of death recorded on hospital charts and those on death certificates revealed the following:

1. The death certificates underestimate birth trauma.
2. The death certificates under-report malformations.
3. There is agreement on infections and anoxia.
4. There is agreement on hemolytic diseases in all categories except C premature infants.

The recording of too few cases of birth trauma on the death certificates is indicative of a tendency to assign cases to unavoidable causes rather than to those which carried an

Table LVII. Percentage Distribution of Perinatal Deaths—
By Causes on Death Certificates

PREMATURE INFANTS

Causes	A	B	C
Birth trauma	2	5	6
Anoxia	46	10	2
Malformations	2	7	7
Infections	1	5	32
Hemolytic diseases	3	2	2
Pulmonary pathology	0	15	8
Prematurity	8	53	41
Unknown and other cause	38	3	2
Total	100	100	100

MATURE INFANTS

Causes	A	B	C
Birth trauma	2	11	1
Anoxia	46	13	3
Malformations	6	24	21
Infections	0	10	47
Hemolytic diseases	4	9	9
Pulmonary pathology	1	26	8
Prematurity	0	1	1
Unknown and other cause	41	6	10
Total	100	100	100

onus. The under-reporting of malformations is probably due to absence of autopsy findings at the time the certificate was signed.

These categories do not take into account the intragroup disagreements. Therefore, a compensation may result; when the cases are grouped into broad categories, agreement as to diagnosis between death certificate and clinical record may appear to be more frequent than it really is.

The correlation tables, in which causes of death were originally recorded, demonstrated that it was possible to assign every death to a specific cause as indicated by autopsy, clinical record, or death certificate. In this way the obscuring of intragroup disagreement was avoided. This is reflected in

Tables LVIII to LXIII, which are based on the original specific data; there is greater discordance among the individual comparisons they present than there would have been if causes had been broadly classified.

The exclusion of prematurity as a cause of death among the causes on the clinical record and the frequency with which prematurity was listed as the cause on the death certificates make comparison of this item from the two sources meaningless. Among the premature infants this cause was recorded on 53 per cent of the B category death certificates and on 41 per cent of the C category death certificates. It even appeared on an occasional death certificate for a mature infant. Prematurity is listed as the cause of death on 8.3 per cent of the stillbirth certificates executed for premature stillborn infants.

A more detailed examination of the causes of death among the premature infants of the B group on whom complete autopsies were performed shows that of four instances of cardiac malformations (autopsy diagnosis), only one was so designated on the death certificate; two were called "prematurity" and one was called "atelectasis."[1]

In 41 deaths attributed to "prematurity" on the death certificates, autopsy revealed the causes listed on page 79.

Thus all these 41 deaths ascribed to prematurity on the death certificate could be classified. Only 4 cases (3 of abruptio placentae and 1 of maternal disease) involved infants whose deaths could not be explained anatomically.

The reason for stating that the clinical causes of death

[1] A specimen of the tabulations on which this discussion is based appears in Appendix II. It is representative of 42 tables on causes of death compiled in the course of the study. The entire body of basic data from which the tables in this book are drawn is on file in the office of the Committee on Public Health Relations of The New York Academy of Medicine.

Tentorial tear with hemorrhage	3
Other cerebral hemorrhage	2
Abruptio placentae	3
Maternal disease	1
Cardiac malformation	2
Genitourinary malformations	1
Pneumonia	1
Septicemia	1
Erythroblastosis	1
Atelectasis with hyaline membranes	11
Atelectasis without hyaline membranes	15
Total	41

were more reliable than the causes on the death certificates will be elaborated in the following section.

AGREEMENT ON CAUSES

Causes from all three sources—clinical, pathologic, and death certificates—have been recorded for each case in the study, and correlations are possible. A "disagreement" is recorded if the sources of information on the causes do not classify the case under the same rubric. Considerable leeway was allowed to take care of conditions impossible to differentiate clinically. For example, a diagnosis on a death certificate of "cardiac anomaly" which on autopsy was found to be pulmonary anomaly was recorded as an agreement.

Tables LVIII through LX demonstrate the degree of agreement for cases in which complete autopsies[2] were performed. The causes on the death certificates and the pathologic causes agreed 40 per cent of the time. The causes on the death certificates and the clinical causes agreed approximately to the

[2] A complete autopsy is understood to be a complete pathologic examination, including examination of the head and microscopic study of the body tissues.

Table LVIII. Percentage of Agreement of Death Certificate and Autopsy Diagnoses—*Complete Autopsies*

	Total No.	*In Agreement* No.	*In Agreement* Per Cent
A			
Premature	6	2	33
Mature	14	7	50
Total A	20	9	45
B*			
Premature	81	19	24
Mature	66	36	55
Total B	147	55	37
C			
Premature	30	11	37
Mature	42	18	43
Total C	72	29	40
A+B+C (adjusted)			
Premature	—	—	28
Mature	—	—	50
Total A+B+C	—	—	40

* Appendix II, "Specimen Correlation Table," shows the basic data from which these B percentages are derived.

Table LIX. Percentage of Agreement of Death Certificate and Clinical Diagnoses—*Complete Autopsies*

	Total No.	*In Agreement* No.	*In Agreement* Per Cent
A			
Premature	6	2	33
Mature	14	5	36
Total A	20	7	35
B			
Premature	81	20	25
Mature	66	40	61
Total B	147	60	41
C			
Premature	30	11	37
Mature	42	22	52
Total C	72	33	46
A+B+C (adjusted)			
Premature	—	—	28
Mature	—	—	55
Total A+B+C	—	—	42

Table LX. Percentage of Agreement of Clinical and Autopsy Diagnoses—*Complete Autopsies*

	Total No.	*In Agreement* No.	*In Agreement* Per Cent
A			
Premature	6	6	100
Mature	14	11	79
Total A	20	17	85
B			
Premature	81	56	69
Mature	66	45	68
Total B	147	101	69
C			
Premature	30	19	63
Mature	42	24	57
Total C	72	43	60
A+B+C (adjusted)			
Premature	—	—	69
Mature	—	—	66
Total A+B+C	—	—	67

same extent, 42 per cent. On the other hand, the clinical causes and the pathologic causes agreed 67 per cent of the time.

It must be borne in mind that "prematurity" was not allowed as a cause of death in the autopsy and clinical diagnoses. Therefore, wherever the diagnosis on the death certificate was "prematurity" there was a disagreement. The magnitude of the difference is explained when it is realized that one-half of the B and C deaths are in this possible category. This is clearly reflected in the extent of agreement for the premature versus the mature infants.

Tables LXI, LXII, and LXIII present corresponding data for the cases in which there were incomplete autopsies. The results show 50 per cent agreement between causes on the death certificates and pathologic causes; 54 per cent agreement between causes on the death certificates and the

Table LXI. Percentage of Agreement of Death Certificate and Pathologic Diagnoses—*Incomplete Autopsies*

	Total	*In Agreement*	
	No.	No.	Per Cent
A			
Premature	13	4	31
Mature	23	16	70
Total A	36	20	56
B			
Premature	43	10	23
Mature	42	25	60
Total B	85	35	41
C			
Premature	16	4	25
Mature	38	28	74
Total C	54	32	59
A+B+C (adjusted)			
Premature	—	—	25
Mature	—	—	67
Total A+B+C	—	—	50

Table LXII. Percentage of Agreement of Death Certificate and Clinical Diagnoses—*Incomplete Autopsies*

	Total	*In Agreement*	
	No.	No.	Per Cent
A			
Premature	13	4	31
Mature	23	14	61
Total A	36	18	50
B			
Premature	43	17	40
Mature	42	28	67
Total B	85	45	53
C			
Premature	16	4	25
Mature	38	28	74
Total C	54	32	59
A+B+C (adjusted)			
Premature	—	—	35
Mature	—	—	68
Total A+B+C	—	—	54

Table LXIII. Percentage of Agreement of Clinical and Pathologic Diagnoses—*Incomplete Autopsies*

	Total No.	*In Agreement* No.	*In Agreement* Per Cent
A			
Premature	13	11	85
Mature	23	18	78
Total A	36	29	81
B			
Premature	43	30	70
Mature	42	32	76
Total B	85	62	73
C			
Premature	16	9	56
Mature	38	29	76
Total C	54	38	70
A+B+C (adjusted)			
Premature	—	—	70
Mature	—	—	77
Total A+B+C	—	—	74

clinical causes; and 74 per cent agreement between clinical causes and pathologic causes.

Thus it is apparent that when an autopsy was performed, either partial or complete, the cause recorded on the death certificate was not made 100 per cent accurate. In fact, the best result, on the whole, was to bring about 50 per cent accuracy.

In an isolated group the result may be better, as in the group of C mature infants with incomplete autopsies, where agreement was 74 per cent. The death certificate does not always utilize the information produced by an autopsy and therefore shows up unfavorably when compared with the pathologic diagnosis obtained at either complete or incomplete autopsy.

The agreement of the clinical and the autopsy diagnoses

Table LXIV. Percentage of Agreement of Death Certificate and Clinical Diagnoses—*Not Autopsied*

	Total No.	*In Agreement* No.	*In Agreement* Per Cent
A			
Premature	91	51	56
Mature	90	48	53
Total A	181	99	55
B			
Premature	155	32	21
Mature	96	42	44
Total B	251	74	30
C			
Premature	41	14	34
Mature	68	41	60
Total C	109	55	51
A+B+C (adjusted)			
Premature	—	—	34
Mature	—	—	52
Total A+B+C	—	—	42

as shown in Tables LX and LXIII may have been influenced by the autopsy findings as recorded.

The clinical causes and the pathologic causes agree about 70 per cent of the time. This agreement varies relatively little between premature and mature infants, category by category, and appears to have been little influenced by the completeness of the autopsies.

The foregoing shows the reasoning which leads to the statement that for this study the clinical cause of death is preferred to the cause recorded on the death certificate.

Table LXIV demonstrates that when autopsy was not performed, the cause entered on the death certificate and the clinical cause agreed 42 per cent of the time.

Table LXV compares the clinical causes of death with the causes on the death certificates for all cases in the study. This reveals an agreement 44 per cent of the time.

Table LXV. Percentage of Agreement of Death Certificate and Clinical Diagnoses—*All Deaths*

	Total No.	*In Agreement* No.	Per Cent
A			
Premature	110	57	52
Mature	127	67	53
Total A	237	124	52
B			
Premature	279	69	25
Mature	204	110	54
Total B	483	179	37
C			
Premature	88	29	33
Mature	147	91	62
Total C	235	120	51
A+B+C (adjusted)			
Premature	—	—	33
Mature	—	—	56
Total A+B+C	—	—	44

From the survey of the cases in which autopsy was performed, it may be concluded that for infants dying in the perinatal period the cause of death recorded on the death certificate is the correct one only 50 per cent of the time. This surprising finding detracts from the value of vital statistics reports prepared from data on death certificates.

An effort was made to ascertain the degree of consistency between the certificates of births, deaths, and stillbirths and the available clinical histories on items other than the causes of death.

All items for category A (stillbirths) were procured from the stillbirth certificates. For categories B and C the source of information was the birth certificate except for the item "autopsy performed," which was obtained from the death certificate.

Table LXVI demonstrates the degree of disagreement be-

Table LXVI. Percentage of Disagreement Between Certificates and Clinical Records—*For 10 Selected Items*

Items	*A*	*B*	*C*	*Adjusted Total*
Age of father	13	15	14	14
Age of mother	3	5	3	4
Operation	21	11	10	16
Duration of pregnancy	62	72	66	66
Maternal complications	25	13	11	19
Rh determination	50	36	41	44
Test for syphilis	21	19	19	20
Fetal position	10	7	7	9
Weight of infant	35	19	13	27
Autopsy performed	10	4	4	7
No. of Deaths	*237*	*483*	*235*	

tween the records for ten selected items. The duration of pregnancy was reported as lacking agreement if the difference between the notations on the clinical record and on the certificate was 8 or more days. The reports on the weight of the infant were regarded as discrepant if the difference in recorded weight was in excess of 50 grams. Statements concerning operations were recorded as inconsistent if there was variance about the type of operation or the performance of an operation. Rh determinations and tests for syphilis were recorded as being in disagreement if there were differences in the results, or if an item appeared on only one record.

The present study records only the presence or absence of disagreement and takes no note of the degree of divergence.

One might question the value of interpretations and tabulations prepared from some of the "supplemental" items on the birth and stillbirth certificates, in view of the data in Table LXVI.

In Table LXVII is recorded the number of disagreements per death and their distribution.

Table LXVII shows that only 6.3 per cent of the cases exhibit no disagreements between the certificates and the clini-

Table LXVII. Percentage Distribution of Perinatal Deaths—
By Number of Certificate Disagreements

Disagreements	*A*	*B*	*C*	*Adjusted Total*
0	4.6	7.9	9.8	6.3
1	20.3	30.2	34.0	25.0
2	26.6	31.7	31.5	28.9
3	26.6	19.0	14.0	22.6
4	16.0	7.9	6.8	12.0
5	3.8	2.1	3.0	3.4
6	1.3	1.0	0.9	1.1
7	0.4	0.2	0.0	0.3
8	0.4	0.0	0.0	0.2
No. of Deaths	*237*	*483*	*235*	
No. of disagreements per patient	2.5	2.0	1.9	2.3

cal history; that is, 93.7 per cent of the cases exhibited one or more disagreements between data as recorded on the certificates and on the clinical record. When it is recalled that the data used in the present section omit any disparities in the recorded causes of death, the differences become even more striking.

A more detailed study of these and other disagreements is contemplated by the author. In this future study an attempt will be made to identify and locate the errors. It is hoped that certain questions may be answered. Who is responsible for the disagreements? Are they of equal frequency in all types of institutions and in all categories of death or birth? Do all types of professional service contribute equally to these inconsistencies?

It must be pointed out that each certificate is signed by a physician who certifies that to the best of his knowledge the information contained thereon is correct.

CHAPTER IX

Summary

A STRATIFIED sample of 955 perinatal deaths was selected from the total number of perinatal deaths of infants of over 1000 grams' birth weight occurring in New York City in the year 1950 and the first quarter of 1951. The clinical records of the babies and their mothers were examined in detail.

On the basis of the analysis, the following conclusions may be drawn concerning the perinatal deaths of New York City for the study period:

1. Thirty-five per cent of the deaths were preventable. Table XIV.

2. The frequency of preventability (preventability rate) for deaths of mature infants was 1.45 times as great as that for the deaths of premature infants. Table XIV.

3. The presence of a responsibility factor other than "unavoidable disaster" was associated with an increase in the rate of preventability. Table XVI.

4. For all the deaths studied (preventable and non-preventable) the responsibility factors most frequently present (based on Table XV) were:

Unavoidable disaster	55 per cent
Errors in medical judgment	31 per cent
Unsatisfactory pediatric care	27 per cent
Errors in medical technique	24 per cent
Faulty prenatal care	22 per cent

5. The house staffs had the highest preventability rate and the obstetricians the lowest. The responsibility factors carrying high preventability rates were recorded with greatest frequency for the house staff and least frequently for the obstetricians. On the other hand, "unavoidable disaster" associated with a negligible preventability rate was recorded most frequently for the obstetricians. Based on Table XXIV.

6. Teaching hospitals enjoyed a lower rate of preventability than did the non-teaching hospitals. The lowest rate was recorded for the voluntary teaching hospitals. Table XXVIII.

7. There were slightly more ward service cases among the perinatal deaths than among total births, a reflection of higher perinatal "mortality rates" for such patients. The preventability "rates" were consistently higher for deaths in ward service cases than for deaths in private cases. Table XX.

8. Conclusions concerning the role of prenatal care cannot be drawn because the extent of such care was unknown in about 40 per cent of the deaths. Table XXI.

9. The following responsibility factors occurred infrequently (Table XXV):

Unqualified medical attendant
Intercurrent infection
Family at fault

10. Thirty-five per cent of the babies (adjusted total) were submitted to either complete or partial necropsy. The highest frequency of autopsies was in the C category, 54 per cent (Table LIII). The performance of autopsies aided in accurate assessment of the cause of death. The performance of an autopsy did not influence the determination of preventability.

11. Previous perinatal loss was greatest among mothers

delivering stillborn infants in the pregnancies under review (A). Table XXXIV.

12. Previous abortions were most frequent among mothers of babies who died in the early neonatal period (B). Table XXXIV.

13. Toxemias of pregnancy were of almost equal frequency among the mothers of the premature and the mature infants. Table XXXV.

14. Stillbirths associated with toxemias of pregnancy carried a preventability rate several times that observed when toxemias were absent. Among the early neonatal deaths the rate was the same regardless of the presence of toxemias of pregnancy. Among the late neonatal deaths the preventability rate was higher for those deaths not associated with toxemias of pregnancy. Table XXXVI.

15. In over 48 per cent of the deaths of premature infants a general anesthetic had been used during the delivery. Table XL.

16. Twenty-eight per cent of the deaths of premature infants and 14 per cent of the deaths of mature infants were associated with abnormal presentations at delivery (page 57).

17. Operative delivery was employed in 46 per cent of the deaths of premature infants and in 52 per cent of the mature infants. Fifteen per cent of the premature babies who died were delivered by cesarean section. Table XLIV.

18. Forty-six per cent of the mature stillborn infants died during labor. Twenty-four per cent of the premature stillbirths occurred during labor. Table XLVI.

19. The preventability rate for infants dying during labor was 35 per cent for the premature and 62 per cent for the mature infants. Table XLVIII.

20. When a complete autopsy had been performed, death certificate diagnoses and autopsy diagnoses agreed only 40 per cent of the time. When an incomplete autopsy had been performed, the agreement was 50 per cent. Tables LVIII and LXI.

21. When a complete autopsy had been performed, the clinical diagnoses and the autopsy diagnoses agreed 67 per cent of the time. When an incomplete autopsy had been performed, the agreement was 74 per cent. Tables LX and LXIII.

22. The death certificate diagnosis and the clinical diagnosis, for all 955 cases, agreed 44 per cent of the time. Table LXV.

23. The clinical causes of death were adjudged to give the best information for the entire series of 955 deaths.

24. For all 955 deaths, data on the birth, death, or stillbirth certificates disagreed appreciably with data on the clinical records for ten selected items (Table LXVI). There were 2.3 disagreements per death. Only 6.3 per cent of the deaths exhibited no disagreements. Table LXVII.

The experience gained in the present study indicates that the following suggestions may be pertinent to similar studies:

1. In order to have a basis for comparison, the field study should include the collection of identical data for three series of infants consisting of some who were stillborn, some who succumbed in the neonatal period, and some who survived the neonatal period.

2. A careful decision must be made as to the categories or subcategories to be studied—stillbirths or the various categories of neonatal deaths; premature or mature infants and the like. If premature infants are to be studied, it is suggested

that the weight range from 1001 grams to 2500 grams be subdivided into smaller categories. The mortality rates vary so widely between these extremes of prematurity, and the importance of antenatal and intrapartum factors varies so greatly from the lower to the upper extremes of prematurity, that placing all these infants in one category makes subsequent evaluations difficult and questionable. The various subgroups need not be sampled in the same proportions. The sampling proportions may be made larger or smaller, depending upon the total number of infants within a subgroup.

3. In order to maintain uniformity of investigation and evaluation, the field workers must be thoroughly trained. The field reports must be carefully checked. It is essential that each record be complete.

4. Since vital statistics records are usually the source of the sample, the sampling procedure must take into account the time schedule of the vital statistics agency. A check must be maintained to assure that each record has the predetermined chance of being chosen.

5. It may not be possible to achieve a city-wide study involving detailed autopsy findings unless the pathologists have been especially oriented to follow a uniform method of procedure and interpretation. In the absence of such a city-wide plan, it may be more profitable to concentrate the study on cases in several institutions where trained pathologists interested in fetal pathology may be willing to adopt uniformity for the period of the study.

6. If preventability is to be determined by a panel, the same panel must pass on all cases and not merely on those selected by an investigator. The panel's decisions should be checked by the resubmission of cases from time to time. This practice will determine what consistency can be expected.

APPENDICES AND REFERENCES

APPENDIX I

Forms Used in the Study

FORM 1. OBSTETRICAL QUESTIONNAIRE

(For Field Team)

CASE NO. . . . . Name: DATE OF DEATH

Age at death . . . .

. . . . Hrs. (If less than 48) Mo. Day Year Hours Am/Pm

. . . . Days (If more than 2)

O– 1. Place of Death: . . . .
(Specify hospital, or street no. if home)

2. Mother's Name . . . .
(Last) (First)

3. Age . . . . . . Color . . . . . . Para . . . . . . Wass. . . . . . . Date . . . . . .
Antiluetic treatment? Yes? No? Adeq.? Inadeq.?
L.M.P. . . . . . .

4. Father's age . . . . . . Color . . . . . . Health . . . . . . RH . . . . . .

5. Mother's RH . . . . . . Anti-RH . . . . . . R.B.C. . . . . Hgb . . . .
Blood Type . . . . . .

6. Baby's RH . . . . . . Cord Wassermann . . . . . .

7. NUMBER OF OTHER CHILDREN
Full-term: Living . . . . . . Dead . . . . . . Stillborn . . . . . . Cause. . . . . .
Premature: Living . . . . . Dead . . . . . . Stillborn . . . . . . Cause . . . . . .
Abortions or miscarriages . . . . . . Cause . . . . Diagnosis . . . .

8. Abnormalities of preceding pregnancies? . . . .

9. Prenatal Visits: . . . . Instruction . . . . Examination? . . . .
(How many, how often, what nature, by whom?)

10. Diet: Proteins abundant? . . . . . . Vitamins? . . . . . . Restricted fluids? . . . . . . Restricted salt? . . . . . .

HISTORY OF PREGNANCY

11. Antepartum Complications (Endocrine, toxemia, etc.) . . . .
(Bacteria and viral infections) . . . .

12. Treatment? . . . .

13. HISTORY OF LABOR:
   a. Complications? .... Consultation? ....
   b. If over 24 hours, was consultant called in?
   c. Was pelvic conformation determined by x-ray examination?
   d. How often was fetal heart auscultated before / after rupture of membranes?
   e. Did mother receive vitamin K during labor?
   f. Did care during labor conform with minimal standards?

HISTORY OF DELIVERY

14. Weeks of gestation ...... presentation ...... maternal condition ...... fetal condition ......
15. Method of delivery ...... Hrs: 1st stage ...... 2nd stage ......
16. Name and title of attendant(s) ....
17. Indications, if operative ....
18. Was labor induced? .... Indications .... Method ....
19. How long were membranes ruptured before labor? .... before delivery? ......
20. Abnormalities of placenta ....
    of cord: prolapse .... knotted .... around neck ....
    of amniotic fluid ....
21. Medication to mother (Dosage ...... Time before actual birth .....)
22. Opium derivative .... Scopolamine .... Barbiturate .... Other ....
23. Anesthesia: (Kind, amount, length of administration before birth) .... By whom administered ....
24. Baby's condition: Color .... Oxygen administered? .... When? ....
25. Breathing begun spontaneously? .... Induced? ....
26. Resuscitation: Type? .... By whom administered? ....
27. Puerperal complications ....

....

Investigator

FORM 2. PEDIATRIC QUESTIONNAIRE

CASE NO. NAME: HOSPITAL HISTORY NO.

Mother's ....
Baby's ....

P– 1. Age at death
...... Days (If more than 2) ...... Hrs. (If less than 48)
Date of death: ....
Mo. Day Year Hour Am/Pm

2. *a.* Place of birth ....
b. Place of death ....
(Specify name of hospital, or street no. if home)
Delivery room ....
Nursery ....

3. Birth weight .... Length ....
Duration of pregnancy .... weeks

4. Color ...... Sex ...... If premature, specify cause of this ....
....
syphilis ....

5. What evidence of birth trauma ....
congenital anomalies ....
Record: Rh ...... Blood type .... Cord Wassermann ....

6. Incubator used? .... When? .... How long? ....

7. Heated crib used? .... When? .... How long? ....

8. If multiple pregnancy, which infant is this? ....

9 *a.* Medical attention by:
Obstetrician ....
Pediatrician ....
Physician ....
Resident staff (specify service) ....
Others (specify)

b. Consultation by .... Date ....
c. Was oxygen administered? .... When? .... How long? ....
d. Was oxygen-carbon dioxide mixture given? ...... When? ......
How long? ....
e. Other medication ....

10. Any symptoms of disease? .... When noted? ....
By whom? ....

11. How transported to nursery? .... When? ....
Type of nursery (ordinary, premature, isolation) ....

12. Initial physical examination in nursery
Admission weight .... Circumf. head .... chest ....
Gen. appearance .... Temp. .... Pallor, cyanosis ....
Icterus ...... Breathing ...... Skin ...... S.C. Tissue ......
Cry ....
HEAD: A.font ...... P.font ...... Sutures .... Eyes ......
Ears ...... Nose ...... Mouth ...... Throat ...... Neck ......
CHEST: Lungs .... Heart .... Murmurs ....
ABDOMEN: Liver .... Spleen .... Kidneys ....
GENITALS: .... ANUS .... SPINE ....

MUSCULAR SYST. . . . .
EXTREMITIES: Reflexes . . . . . . Joints . . . . . . Moro . . . .

13. Feeding Date Constituents Amount Frequency Method
Initial (hr.) . . . .
Subsequent (days) . . . .
. . . .
. . . .
. . . .

14. Supplements

Vitamin	Preparation	Date	Hr. begun	Dosage	Route	Changes
K						
C						
A						
D						
(others)						
Iron						

15. Course Dates Description
Abnorm. Temp. . . . .
Apnœa . . . .
Cyanosis . . . .
Resp. infect. . . . .
Diarrhea . . . .
Vomiting . . . .
Convulsions . . . .
Cerebral hem. . . . .
Jaundice . . . .
Hemorrhage . . . .
Malformations . . . .
Other conditions . . . .

16. Significant laboratory and/or x-ray data . . . .
. . . .

17. Treatment

Treatment	Dates	Amount	Route	Frequency	Indications
Clysis	. . . . .	. . . .	. . . . .	. . . .	. . . .
Infusion	. . . . .	. . . .	. . . . .	. . . .	. . . .
Blood	. . . . .	. . . .	. . . . .	. . . .	. . . .
Sulfa	. . . . .	. . . .	. . . . .	. . . .	. . . .
Penicillin	. . . . .	. . . .	. . . . .	. . . .	. . . .
Streptomycin	. . . . .	. . . .	. . . . .	. . . .	. . . .
Others	. . . . .	. . . .	. . . . .	. . . .	. . . .

. . . .
Investigator

Form 3. PATHOLOGY QUESTIONNAIRE

CASE NO. .... NAME ....
Was autopsy performed? .... By whom? ....
Title of pathologist ....
Certified by Am. Bd. Path.? ....
Was autopsy complete? ...... Restricted? ...... Cultures taken? ......
From what organs taken? ....
Was skull opened? .... Brain sectioned? ....
Were microscopic sections made? .... Described? ....
Was pulmonary tissue examined microscopically? ....
Cause of death ....
Contributing factors ....
Anatomic pathologic diagnosis ....

....
Investigator

Form 4. SUMMARY SHEET

CASE NO.

NEW YORK ACADEMY OF MEDICINE
SUBCOMMITTEE ON NEONATAL MORTALITY
STUDY OF NEONATAL MORTALITY

COMMITTEE OPINION
Primary ....
Secondary ....

NAME PLACE OF DEATH ADDRESS OF MOTHER

DATE OF DEATH .... 19......
Mo. Day Year
.... A.M. .... Hrs. (if less than 48)
.... P.M. .... Days (if more than two)
AUTOPSY? BY WHOM? TITLE
CAUSE OF DEATH Immediate .... Contributing ....
ATTENDING PHYSICIAN(S) .... THEIR TITLES ....
STAFF OPINION ....
I II III A B Hospital rating:

1 2 3 4 5 6 7 STUDY FORM FILLED OUT BY:
COMMITTEE COMMENTS ....

FORM 5. CODE SHEET

PERINATAL MORTALITY (SPECIAL) NAME . . . .

Case Number
1 2-3 4

COL. 5–6. Hospital—Delivery

COL. 7. Borough of Residence (S. F.)
0. Same as birth
1. Manhattan
2. Bronx
3. Brooklyn
4. Queens
5. Staten Island

COL. 7. Consultations
6. Medical
7. Obstetrical
8. Surgical
9. Gynecological

COL. 8. Month of Death

COL. 9. Age of Mother
0. Less than 15
1. 15–19
2. 20–24
3. 25–29
4. 30–34
5. 35–39
6. 40–44
7. 45–49
8. 50 and over
Y. Unknown

COL. 10. Age of Father

COL. 11. Race-Social Status
0. Colored Ward Married
1. Colored Ward Unmarried
2. Colored Private Married
3. Colored Private Unmarried
4. Colored Ward Unknown
5. White Ward Married
6. White Ward Unmarried
7. White Private Married
8. White Private Unmarried
9. White Ward Unknown
X. Other Married
Y. Other Unmarried

COL. 12. Prenatal Care (S. F.) (PMP)
0. None
1. 1–3 visits
2. 4–8 visits
3. 9 or more visits
4. Hospital Dispensary
5. Other Dispensary
6. Private obstetrician
7. Private physician (not obstetrician)
8. Inertia
9. Pelvic dystocia
X. Other dystocia
Y. Unknown

COL. 13. Pelvis
0. None listed
1. Normal
2. Contracted inlet
3. Midpelvic contraction
4. Outlet contraction
5. Inlet and outlet contraction
6. Inlet and midplane contraction
7. Midplane and outlet contraction
8. Inlet-outlet and midplane contraction
9. Asymmetrical contraction
X. Other abnormalities
Y. Unknown

COL. 14. Full term Preg.

COL. 15. Premature Preg.

COL. 16. Abortions

COL. 17. Living children

COL. 18. Previous Stillbirths S.F.
0. None
1. One
2. Two
3. Three
4. Four
5. Five or more

COL. 18. Previous Neonatal Deaths
6. None
7. One
8. Two
9. Three
X. Four
Y. Five or more

COL. 19. Preg. Fol. PMP
0. None
1. Acute toxemia
2. Chronic toxemia
3. Renal disease
4. Heart disease without failure
5. Heart disease with failure
6. Tuberculosis
7. Isoimmunization
8. Diabetes
9. Mole or chorio
X. Other

COL. 20. Fetal Heart on Adm. to Hosp. (S.F.) (PMP)
0. Not recorded
1. Absent
2. Questionable
3. Present—good
4. Present—poor
5. Rate less than 100
6. Rate greater than 180
7. Rate less than 80
X. Intrapartum
Y. Antepartum

COL. 21. Toxemia (S.F.)
0. No toxemia
1. Eclampsia, antepartum
2. Eclampsia, intrapartum
3. Preeclampsia
4. Hypertensive disease
5. Unclassified
6. Alb. present—A.P.
7. Alb. present—I.P.
8. Alb. unknown

COL. 22. Dis. of this Preg. (1)
0. None listed
1. Pulmonary tbc. active
2. Pulmonary tbc. inactive
3. Tbc. elsewhere
4. Other pulmonary disease
5. Thyroid—Hyper.
6. Thyroid—Hypo.
7. Diabetes
8. Liver disease
9. Respiratory disease
X. Heart disease—failure
Y. Heart disease—no failure

COL. 23. Dis. of this Preg. (2)
0. None listed
1. Rubella
2. Other virus disease
3. First trimester
4. Second trimester
5. Mechanical trauma
6. Pyelitis
7. Other urinary tract infection
8. Acute infectious disease
9. Myoma
X. Threatened abortion
Y. Other significant disease

COL. 24. Rh Mother
0. None listed
1. Rh positive
2. Rh neg.—sensitized
3. Rh neg.—not sensitized
4. Rh neg.—sensit. unknown
5. Other isoimmunization

COL. 24. Rh Baby
6. None listed
7. Rh positive
8. Rh negative
9. Rh unknown
X. Coombs—negative
Y. Coombs—positive

COL. 25. Venereal Disease (S.F.)
0. None listed
1. S.T.S. negative
2. S.T.S. positive—untreated
3. S.T.S. positive—treated
4. Previous syphilis
5. S.T.S. not taken
6. Gonorrhea
7. Lymphopathia
8. Other venereal disease

COL. 25. Anemia
9. Anemia treated
X. Anemia untreated
Y. Anemia treatment unknown

COL. 26. Weight Gain of Mother
0. Less than 10 pounds
9. 90 plus pounds
X. Loss of weight
Y. Weight gain unknown

COL. 27. Period of Gestation
0. Less than 28 weeks
1. 28–29 weeks
2. 30–31
3. 32–33
4. 34–35
5. 36–37
6. 38–39
7. 40–41
8. 42–43
9. 44–45
X. 46 plus weeks
Y. Unknown

COL. 28. Presentation
0. Vertex anterior
1. Vertex posterior
2. Vertex rotated
3. Breech frank
4. Breech full
5. Breech footling
6. Face or brow
7. Compound
8. Transverse lie
9. Multiple pregnancy
Y. Unknown

COL. 29. Int. between fetal death & onset of labor (S.F.)
0. Alive at onset
1. Less than 24 hours
2. 24–48 hrs.
3. 49–72 hrs.
4. 3–8 days
5. 9–12 days
6. 13–29 days
7. 30 or more days
8. Unknown

COL. 29. Birth order
X. First child
Y. Second child

COL. 30. Labor Onset PMP
0. None listed
1. Spontaneous
2. Strip. memb., successful
3. Strip. memb., unsuccessful
4. Rupture of membranes successful
5. Rupture of membranes, unsuccessful
6. Drug successful
7. Drug unsuccessful
8. Other
Y. Unknown

COL. 31. Membranes Rupt. PMP
0. Membranes ruptured spontaneously
1. Membranes ruptured artificially
2. LP less than 2 hrs.
3. LP 2–12 hrs.
4. LP more than 12 hrs.
5. LP unknown
6. Less than 24 hrs. to delivery
7. More than 24 hrs. to delivery
8. Before 5 cms.
9. 5–10 cms.
X. Turbidity of amniotic fluid
Y. Unknown

COL. 32. Indications for Rupt. of Membranes
0. Not ruptured artificially
1. Induce labor—convenience

(continued on next page)

COL. 32 (cont.)
2. Induce labor obstetrical indication
3. Induce labor medical indication
4. Speed labor—convenience
5. Speed labor obstetrical indication
6. Speed labor medical indication
7. Inertia—primary
8. Inertia—secondary

COL. 33. Time Int. from Disap. of Fetal Heart to Del.
0. Present at delivery
1. Less than 30 min.
2. 30–60 min.
3. 61–90 min.
4. 91–120 min.
5. 121–180 min.
6. 181–220 min.
7. 221–260 min.
8. Over 260 min.
9. Slowing of fetal heart in labor
X. Second stage
Y. Unknown

COL. 34. Duration—First Stage
0. None
1. Less than 5 hrs.
2. 5–9
3. 10–14
4. 15–19
5. 20–24
6. 25–29
7. 30–39
8. 40 and over
Y. Unknown

COL. 35. Dur. of 2nd Stage (PMP)
0. None
1. Less than 60 min.
2. 60–119
3. 120–179
4. 180–239
5. 240–299
6. 5 hours and over
9. Total labor greater than 24 hrs.
X. Total labor greater than 30 hrs.
Y. Unknown

COL. 36. Labor Compl. (1)
0. None listed
1. Placenta previa total
2. Placenta previa partial
3. Placenta low implanted
4. Placenta—premature separation
5. Rupture marginal sinus
6. Rupture of uterus
7. Other antepartum hemorrhage
8. Prolapse of cord
9. Cephalopelvic disproportion
X. Abnormal contraction
Y. Cervical dystocia

COL. 37. Labor Compl. (2)
0. None listed
1. Intrapartum fever
2. Uterine inertia, primary
3. Uterine inertia, secondary
4. Shock
5. Anesthetic accident
6. Cerebral accident
7. Shoulder dystocia
8. Hydrocephalus
9. Other fetal dystocia
X. Father Rh negative
Y. Father Rh positive

COL. 38. Type of Delivery
0. Spont. without episiotomy
1. Spont. with episiotomy
2. Low forceps
3. Mid forceps
4. High forceps
5. Destructive operation
6. Section
7. Version
8. Breech, spont.
9. Breech, extraction
X. Elective
Y. Unknown

COL. 39. Analgesia
0. None listed
1. Psychosomatic
2. Barbiturate
3. Morphine and substitutes
4. Paraldehyde
5. Amnesics
6. Conduction
7. Inhalation
8. Other
Y. Unknown

COL. 40. Int.—Last Analgesic to Delivery

0. No analgesia
1. Less than 30 min.
2. 30–59
3. 60–89
4. 90–119
5. 120–149
6. 150–179
7. 180–209
8. 210–239
9. 240–299
X. 3 or plus
Y. Unknown

COL. 41. Anesthesia PMP

0. None listed
1. Inhalation
2. Intravenous
3. Conduction epidural
4. Conduction caudal
5. Conduction saddle
6. Conduction spinal
7. Local
8. Continuous
9. Other
Y. Unknown

COL. 42. Time of Death

0. Died before labor
1. Died during labor
2. Died first 12 hrs.
3. Died 12–24 hrs.
4. Died 24–48 hrs.
5. Died 48–72 hrs.
6. Died 3–10 days
7. Died 10–30 days
8. Died over 30 days
9. Autopsy, complete
X. Male
Y. Autopsy, incomplete

COL. 43. Birth Weight

0. Under 400 gms.
1. 400–999 gms.
2. 1000–1499 gms.
3. 1500–1999 gms.
4. 2000–2499 gms.
5. 2500–2999 gms.
6. 3000–3499 gms.
7. 3500–3999 gms.
8. 4000–4499 gms.
9. 4500–4999 gms.
X. 5000 and over
Y. Unknown

COL. 44. Breathing Time

0. Stillborn
1. Less than 5 seconds
2. 5–29 seconds
3. 30–60 seconds
4. 1–2 minutes
5. 2–3 minutes
6. 3–4 minutes
7. 4–5 minutes
8. 5–10 minutes
9. Over 10 minutes
Y. Unknown

COL. 45–46. Clin. Cause of Death

COL. 47–48. Pathological Classif.

COL. 49–50. Factors in Perinatal Mortality

COL. 51. Preventability

0. Unpreventable
1. Preventable
2. Doubtfully Preventable
3. Unclassified

COL. 51. Responsibility

4. Inadequate prenatal care
5. Family at fault
6. Error in medical judgment
7. Error in medical technique
8. Intercurrent infection
9. Unavoidable disaster
X. Unqualified medical attendant

COL. 52. Father's Occupation

0. None listed
1. Skilled laborer
2. Unskilled laborer
3. White collar worker
4. Proprietor
5. Professional
6. Executive
7. Government
Y. Unknown

COL. 53. Child's Condition at Birth (S.F.)
0. Stillborn
1. Good
2. Cyanotic
3. Flaccid
4. Apneic

COL. 53. Resuscitation
5. Incubator
6. Oxygen-free
7. Oxygen-pressure
8. Aspiration
9. Laryngoscopy
X. Bronchoscopy
Y. Drugs

COL. 54. Medical Care of Infant
0. None
1. Physician—Ped.
2. Physician—Obst.
3. Physician—Other
4. House staff—Ped.
5. House staff—Obst.
6. House staff—Other
7. Nurses only
8. Consultation held
X. Care adequate
Y. Care inadequate

COL. 55 Feeding (S.F.)
0. Stillbirth
1. Breast
2. Mixed
3. Artificial

COL. 55. Vitamin K
4. Mother given Vit. K (oral)
5. Mother given Vit. K (hypo)
6. Mother not given Vit. K
7. Mother Unknown if Vit. K given
8. Baby given Vit. K

COL. 56. Treatment of baby
0. None
1. Clysis
2. Infusion
3. Blood
4. Chemotherapy
5. Antibiotics
6. Respiratory stimulants
Y. Stillbirth

COL. 57. Findings (Baby)
0. None
1. Elevated temperature
2. Apnea
3. Cyanosis
4. Respiratory infection
5. Diarrhea
6. Vomiting
7. Convulsions
8. Jaundice
9. Hemorrhage
Y. Stillborn

COL. 58. Placenta—Wght. (S.F.)
0. No record
1. 400 gms. or less
2. 400–599 gms.
3. 600–799 gms.
4. 800–999 gms.
5. 1000 and over

COL. 58. Placenta—Ratio
6. 1:2 or less
7. 1:2–1:49
8. 1:50–1:69
9. 1:70–1:89
X. 1:90–1:99
Y. Over 1:100

COL. 59. Pathology
0. None
1. Hydrops
2. Large liver
3. Large heart
4. Large adrenals
5. Exchange transfusion
6. Other transfusion
7. Kernicterus
8. Jaundice
9. Anemia
X. Abnormal erythropoiesis
Y. Eosinophilic infiltration

COL. 60. G.I. Tract Pathology
0. None
1. Esophagus—congestion
2. Esophagitis
3. Esophagus—malformation
4. Esophagus—perforation
5. Stomach—erosion or ulcer
6. Gastritis

(continued on next page)

COL. 60 (cont.)
7. Stomach—focal hemorrhage
8. Stomach—malformation
9. Stomach—perforation
X. Intestine—focal hemorrhage
Y. Intestine—enteritis

COL. 61. G.I. Tract
0. None
1. Intestine, obstruction, intrinsic
2. Intestine, obstruction, extrinsic
3. Intestine, perforation
4. Intestine, other malformation

COL. 61. Urinary Passages
5. Ureter, obst., dilated
6. Ureter, not obst., dilated
7. Ureter, other malformation
8. Bladder, inflammation
9. Bladder, malfunction
X. Bladder, malformation
Y. Urethra, any abnormality

COL. 62. Kidney
0. None
1. Congestion
2. Thrombosis of vessels
3. Focal hemorrhage
4. Casts
5. Cysts
6. Polycystic
7. Hypoplastic
8. Dystopia or fused
9. Hydronephrosis
X. Glomerulosclerosis
Y. Other

COL. 63. Lymphoid Tissue
0. None
1. Spleen—enlarged
2. Spleen—ruptured
3. Spleen—large follicles
4. Thymus, large
5. Thymus, involuted
6. Thymus, petechiae
7. Thymus, liquefaction
8. Lymph nodes, subcut.
9. Lymph nodes, thorax
X. Lymph nodes, abdomen
Y. Other

COL. 64. Brain
0. Not examined
1. Congestion
2. Focal subarachnoid hemorrhage
3. Subependymal hemorrhage
4. Other focal cerebral hemorrhage
5. Thrombosis
6. Intraventricular hemorrhage
7. Degeneration
8. Malformation
9. Meningitis
X. Other
Y. Normal

COL. 65. Spinal Cord
0. Not examined
1. Malformations
2. Meningitis
3. Kernicterus
4. Other
5. Normal

COL. 65. Pituitary and Thyroid
6. Not examined
7. Hypoplasia
8. Absence
9. Other
X. Normal
Y. Thyroid abnormality

COL. 66. Genitalia
0. Not examined
1. Hyperemia, gonad.
2. Hyperemia, other genitalia
3. Hemorrhage, gonad.
4. Hemorrhage, other genitalia
5. Ovarian cyst
6. Absence of organs
7. Hypoplasia of organs
8. Hyperplasia of organs
9. Intersexuality
X. Other malformation
Y. Normal

COL. 67. Heart
0. None
1. Petechiae, epicardium
2. Petechiae, endo-myocard.
3. Dilatation

(*continued on next page*)

COL. 67 (cont.)
4. Fatty metamorphosis
5. Hypertrophy without malformation
6. Coronary art. necrosis
7. Coronary art. other path.
8. Fibroelastosis
9. Major malformation
X. Minor malformations
Y. Malformation of aorta, ductus, etc.

COL. 68. Lungs (1)
0. None listed
1. Pleura, petechiae
2. Pleuritis
3. Pneumothorax
4. Interstitial emphysema
5. Mucus in bronchi
6. Bronchitis
7. Immature
8. Hypoplasia
9. Other malformations
X. Severe congestion
Y. Edema fluid—alveoli

COL. 69. Lungs (2)
0. None listed
1. Atelectasis, diffuse
2. Atelectasis, focal
3. Aspiration of amniotic fluid
4. Aspiration of vernix
5. Hyaline membranes
6. Bronchopneumonia
7. Blood in alveoli
8. Interstitial pneumonia
9. Aeration, none
X. Aeration, little
Y. Aeration, much

COL. 70. Liver (1)
0. None
1. Congestion
2. Hematomata
3. Rupture
4. Cloudy swelling
5. Fatty
6. Focal necrosis
7. Right>left
8. Jaundice
9. Hemosiderosis
X. Abnormality of biliary apparatus
Y. Other

COL. 71. Liver (2)
0. Syphilis
1. Cirrhosis

COL. 71. Pancreas
2. None
3. Edema
4. Hemorrhage
5. Inflammation
6. Large islets
7. Necrosis of islets
8. Cystic fibrosis
9. Syphilis
X. Malformations

COL. 72. Adrenal
0. None
1. Hypoplastic
2. Enlarged
3. Congestion, moderate
4. Congestion, severe
5. Focal necrosis
6. Hemorrhage, focal
7. Hemorrhage, severe
8. Lacerations
9. Thrombosed vessels
Y. Other

COL. 73. Skin
0. None
1. Edema
2. Petechiae
3. Presenting part
4. Mammary glands, large
5. Inflammation
6. Scleroderma
7. Malformation
8. Trauma
9. Vernix, white
X. Vernix, yellow
Y. Other

COL. 74–75. Certificate Cause of Death—Primary

COL. 76–77. Certificate Cause of Death—Secondary

COL. 78. Certif. Disagreement
0. None
1. Age Father
2. Age Mother
3. Operation
4. Duration of Pregnancy
5. Maternal Complications
6. Rh
7. S.T.S.
8. Position
9. Weight of Infant
X. Autopsy

COL. 79. Transferred To
0. Not transferred
1. Babies Hospital
2. New York Hospital
3. Harlem Hospital
4. Queens General Hospital
5. St. Vincent's Hospital
6. Flushing Hospital
7. Bellevue Hospital
8. Lincoln Hospital
X. Other municipal
Y. Other voluntary

APPENDIX II

Specimen Correlation Table

CAUSES OF DEATH

COMPLETE AUTOPSIES

B PREMATURES

	PATHOLOGIC CAUSES																	
Death Certificate Causes	*Tent. Tear*	*Subdural*	*Subarach.*	*Abruptio*	*Mat. Disease*	*Cardiac Malf.*	*G.U. Malf.*	*Multiple Malf.*	*G. I. Malf.*	*Pneumonia*	*Septicemia*	*Erythroblastosis*	*Hem. Dis. N.B.*	*Aspiration*	*Atelect. With*	*Atelect. Without*	*Unknown*	*Total*
I.C. Hem.	2														2			4
Subarach.			2															2
Anoxia							1		1				1					3
Asphyxia														2				2
Cardiac Malf.						1												1
Prematurity	3	1	1	3	1	2	1			1	1	1			11	15		41
Pneumonia										1					2	1		4
Peritonitis									1									1
Erythroblast.												1						1
Aspiration														1				1
Atelectasis	1					1	1	1		2			1	1	4	6		18
Other												1			1	1		3
Total	6	1	3	3	1	4	3	1	2	4	1	3	2	4	20	23	0	81

References

1. BUNDESEN, H. Natal Day Deaths. *J.A.M.A.*, 1953, Vol. 153, No. 5, pp. 466–473.
2. BUNDESEN, H. et al. Progress in the Prevention of Needless Neonatal Deaths. *Annual Report of Chicago Health Department,* 1951.
3. DEPARTMENT OF HEALTH, NEW YORK CITY. Personal communications.
4. ———. *Reports,* 1941–1948. City of New York.
5. ———. *City of New York Vital Statistics,* 1950.
6. DEPARTMENT OF OBSTETRICS AND GYNECOLOGY, STATE UNIVERSITY OF NEW YORK, COLLEGE OF MEDICINE, BROOKLYN. *Obstetrical Reports,* 1951, 1952, 1953.
7. D'ESOPO, D. A. A Review of Cesarean Section at Sloane Hospital for Women, 1942–1947. *Am. J. Obst. and Gynec.*, 1950, 59:77.
8. EASTMAN, N. J. *Obstetrics,* 10th ed. Appleton-Century-Crofts, Inc., New York, 1950.
9. GAUSS, C. J. Geburten im kunstlichen Dämmerschlaf. *Arch. f. Gynäk.*, 1906, 78:579.
10. HELLMAN, L. M., and HINGSON, R. A. The Effect of Various Methods of Obstetric Pain Relief on Infant Mortality. *N.Y. State J. of Med.*, 1953, 53:2767.
11. LULL, C. B., and HINGSON, R. A. *Control of Pain in Childbirth,* 3rd ed. J.B. Lippincott Co., Philadelphia, 1948.
12. METROPOLITAN LIFE INSURANCE CO. The Hazardous First Month of Life. *Statistical Bulletin,* 1952, 33:1.
13. NEW YORK ACADEMY OF MEDICINE. *Infant and Maternal Care in New York City.* Columbia University Press, New York, 1952.
14. POTTER, E. L. *Pathology of the Fetus and Newborn.* The Year Book Publishers, Chicago, 1952.
15. SIMPSON, J. Y. On the Employment of the Inhalation of Sulphuric Ether in the Practice of Midwifery. *Month. J. Med. Sc.*, 1847, 7:721.
16. STEINBUCKEL, quoted by Eastman (see 8 above), p. 423.
17. YERUSHALMY, J. et al. Studies in Childbirth Mortality I. *Pub. Health Reports,* 1940, 55:1010.

18. ———. Studies in Childbirth Mortality II. *Pub. Health Reports,* 1940, 55:1195.
19. ———. Studies in Childbirth Mortality III. *Pub. Health Reports,* 1941, 56:1463.

Bei Fragen zur Produktsicherheit wenden Sie sich bitte an:
If you have any questions regarding product safety,
please contact:

Walter de Gruyter GmbH
Genthiner Straße 13
10785 Berlin
productsafety@degruyterbrill.com